Root Caries: From Prevalence to Therapy

Monographs in Oral Science

Vol. 26

Series Editors

A. Lussi Bern
M.A.R. Buzalaf Bauru

Root Caries: From Prevalence to Therapy

Volume Editor

Marcela Rocha de Olivera Carrilho São Paulo

41 figures, 31 in color, and 16 tables, 2017

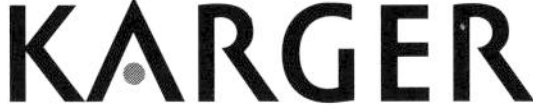

Basel · Freiburg · Paris · London · New York · Chennai · New Delhi · Bangkok · Beijing · Shanghai · Tokyo · Kuala Lumpur · Singapore · Sydney

Marcela Rocha de Olivera Carrilho
Anhanguera University of São Paulo
Biomaterials and Biotechnology &
Innovation in Health Programs
Vila Madalena
Rua Girassol, 584, ap 301A
São Paulo, SP 05433-001 (Brazil)

Library of Congress Cataloging-in-Publication Data

Names: Carrilho, Marcela Rocha de Olivera, editor.
Title: Root caries : from prevalence to therapy / volume editor, Marcela Rocha de Olivera Carrilho.
Other titles: Monographs in oral science ; v. 26. 0077-0892
Description: Basel ; New York : Karger, 2017. | Series: Monographs in oral science, ISSN 0077-0892 ; Vol. 26 | Includes bibliographical references and indexes.
Identifiers: LCCN 2017038123| ISBN 9783318061123 (hard cover : alk. paper) | ISBN 9783318061130 (electronic version)
Subjects: | MESH: Root Caries
Classification: LCC RK331 | NLM WU 270 | DDC 617.6/7--dc23 LC record available at https://lccn.loc.gov/2017038123

Bibliographic Indices. This publication is listed in bibliographic services, including Current Contents® and Index Medicus.

www.karger.com
Printed on acid-free and non-aging paper (ISO 9706)
ISSN 0077–0892
e-ISSN 1662–3843
ISBN 978–3–318–06112–3
e-ISBN 978–3–318–06113–0

Contents

List of Contributors

Patrick Finbarr Allen
Faculty of Dentistry, National University of Singapore
11 Lower Kent Ridge Road
Singapore 119083 (Singapore)
E-Mail denpfa@nus.edu.sg

Luana Severo Alves
Department of Restorative Dentistry, School of Dentistry
Federal University of Santa Maria
Rua Floriano Peixoto, 1184
Santa Maria, RS 97015-372 (Brazil)
E-Mail luanaseal@gmail.com

Avijit Banerjee
King's College London Dental Institute
Floor 26, Tower Wing, Guy's Dental Hospital
Great Maze Pond
London SE1 9RT (UK)
E-Mail avijit.banerjee@kcl.ac.uk

Ana K. Bedran-Russo
Department of Restorative Dentistry
University of Illinois at Chicago
College of Dentistry
801 S. Paulina Street, Room 531a
Chicago, IL 60612 (USA)
E-Mail bedran@uic.edu

Tchilalo Boukpessi
Dental School, University Paris Descartes
1, rue Maurice Arnoux
FR–92120 Montrouge (France)
E-Mail tchilalo.boukpessi@parisdescartes.fr

Francis M. Burke
Restorative Dentistry, Cork University Dental School and Hospital
University College Cork, Wilton
Cork T12 E8YV (Ireland)
E-Mail F.Burke@ucc.ie

Michael Francis Burrow
Faculty of Dentistry
The University of Hong Kong
Prince Philip Dental Hospital
34 Hospital Road
Sai Ying Pun, Hong Kong (SAR China)
E-Mail mfburr58@hku.hk

Marília Afonso Rabelo Buzalaf
Department of Biological Sciences
Bauru School of Dentistry, University of São Paulo
Al. Octávio Pinheiro Brisolla, 9-75
Bauru, SP 17012-901 (Brazil)
E-Mail mbuzalaf@fob.usp.br

Marcela Rocha de Olivera Carrilho
Anhanguera University of São Paulo
Biomaterials and Biotechnology & Innovation in Health Programs
Vila Madalena
Rua Girassol, 584, ap 301A
São Paulo, SP 05433-001 (Brazil)
E-Mail marcelacarrilho@gmail.com

Thiago Saads Carvalho
Department of Preventive, Restorative and Pediatric Dentistry
University of Bern
Freiburgstrasse 7
CH–3010 Bern (Switzerland)
E-Mail thiago.saads@zmk.unibe.ch

Catherine Chaussain
EA 2496, Orofacial Pathologies, Imaging and Biotherapies, Dental School
University Paris Descartes
1, rue Maurice Arnoux
FR–92120 Montrouge (France)
E-Mail catherine.chaussain@parisdescartes.fr

Nailê Damé-Teixeira
Department of Dentistry, Faculty of Health Science,
University of Brasilia
Campus Universitário Darcy Ribeiro
Asa Norte, Brasilia, DF 70910-900 (Brazil)
E-Mail nailedame@hotmail.com

Juliana de Geus
Paulo Picanço Faculty, Rua Joaquim Sa
900 – Dionisio Torres
Fortaleza, CE 60135-218 (Brazil)
E-Mail ju_degeus@hotmail.com

Thuy Do
Division of Oral Biology, School of Dentistry
University of Leeds
Wellcome Trust Brenner Building
St. James University Hospital
Beckett Street
Leeds LS9 7TF (UK)
E-Mail n.t.do@leeds.ac.uk

Sophie Doméjean
UFR d'Odontologie
2, rue de Braga
FR-63100 Clermont-Ferrand (France)
E-Mail sophie.domejean@uca.fr

Ole Fejerskov
Department of Biomedicine
Faculty of Health, Aarhus University
Wilhelm Meyers Allé 3
DK–8000 Aarhus (Denmark)
E-Mail of@biomed.au.dk

Martina Hayes
Restorative Dentistry, Cork University Dental School
and Hospital
University College Cork, Wilton
Cork T12 E8YV (Ireland)
E-Mail Martina.Hayes@ucc.ie

Alessandro D. Loguercio
Department of Restorative Dentistry
State University of Ponta Grossa, Paraná
Av. Carlos Cavalcanti, 4748
Ponta Grossa, PR 84030-900 (Brazil)
E-Mail aloguercio@hotmail.com

Adrian Lussi
Department of Preventive, Restorative and
Pediatric Dentistry
University of Bern
Freiburgstrasse 7
CH–3010 Bern (Switzerland)
E-Mail adrian.lussi@zmk.unibe.ch

Ana Carolina Magalhães
Department of Biological Sciences
Bauru School of Dentistry, University of São Paulo
Al. Octávio Pinheiro Brisolla, 9-75
Bauru, SP 17012-901 (Brazil)
E-Mail acm@fob.usp.br

Marisa Maltz
Department of Social and Preventive Dentistry
Faculty of Odontology
Federal University of Rio Grande do Sul
Rua Ramiro Barcelos, 2492
Porto Alegre, RS 90035-003 (Brazil)
E-Mail marisa.maltz@gmail.com

Philip D. Marsh
Division of Oral Biology, School of Dentistry
University of Leeds
Wellcome Trust Brenner Building
St. James University Hospital
Beckett Street
Leeds LS9 7TF (UK)
E-Mail p.d.marsh@leeds.ac.uk

Suzanne Menashi
EA 2496, Orofacial Pathologies, Imaging and
Biotherapies, Dental School
University Paris Descartes
1, rue Maurice Arnoux
FR–92120 Montrouge (France)
E-Mail suzanne.menashi@gmail.com

Monika Naginyte
Division of Oral Biology, School of Dentistry
University of Leeds
Wellcome Trust Brenner Building
St. James University Hospital
Beckett Street
Leeds LS9 7TF (UK)
E-Mail naginyte@gmail.com

Bente Nyvad
Department of Dentistry and Oral Health
Faculty of Health, Aarhus University
Vennelyst Boulevard 9
DK–8000 Aarhus (Denmark)
E-Mail nyvad@odont.au.dk

Clarissa Cavalcanti Fatturi Parolo
Faculty of Odontology
Federal University of Rio Grande do Sul
Rua Ramiro Barcelos, 2492
Porto Alegre, RS 90035-003 (Brazil)
E-Mail fatturiparolo@yahoo.com

Juliano Pelim Pessan
Department of Pediatric Dentistry and Public Health
School of Dentistry, Araçatuba
São Paulo State University (Unesp)
Rua José Bonifácio, 1193
Araçatuba, SP 16015-050 (Brazil)
E-Mail jpessan@foa.unesp.br

Iain A. Pretty
Dental Health Unit
The University of Manchester
Williams House, Manchester Science Park
Manchester M16 6SE (UK)
E-Mail iain.pretty@manchester.ac.uk

Alessandra Reis
Ponta Grossa State University
Dentistry
Av. Carlos Cavalcanti, 4748
Ponta Grossa, PR 84030-900 (Brazil)
E-Mail reis_ale@hotmail.com

Paulo Vinicius Soares
School of Dentistry, Federal University of Uberlândia
Av. Pará, 1720 – Umuarama
Uberlândia, MG 38405-320 (Brazil)
E-Mail dentistica@umuarama.ufu.br

Margaret A. Stacey
Melbourne Dental School
The University of Melbourne
720 Swanson Street
Carlton, VIC 3010 (Australia)
E-Mail mastacey@unimelb.edu.au

Leo Tjäderhane
Department of Oral and Maxillofacial Diseases
University of Helsinki
PO Box 41
FIN-00014 University of Helsinki (Finland)
E-Mail Leo.Tjaderhane@helsinki.fi

Camila A. Zamperini
University of Illinois at Chicago
College of Dentistry
Department of Restorative Dentistry
801 S. Paulina Street
Chicago, IL 60612 (USA)
E-Mail cazamp82@uic.edu

Julio Eduardo do Amaral Zenkner
Department of Stomatology, School of Dentistry
Federal University of Santa Maria
Rua Floriano Peixoto, 1184
Santa Maria, RS 97015-372 (Brazil)
E-Mail jezenkner@gmail.com

Foreword

It is not very common in the academic life to have the pleasure and opportunity to write a Foreword for such an important and timely publication as "Root Caries: From Prevalence to Therapy." Only yesterday, I was treating a lovely elderly lady with severe root caries problem in and under her otherwise well-functioning bridgework. While trying hard to save her functioning and esthetic occlusion, I could not help but think – again – how difficult and devastating the final outcome of the root caries can be to the patient.

Is this book really timely as I claimed above? Absolutely! For example, just a few months ago, the President of the IADR, Professor Angus Walls titled his IADR 2017 congress opening ceremony speech "Aging – A Call to Arms!" [1]. In his speech, he addressed the challenges posed by the progressive global aging of society and not surprisingly, clearly pointed out that root caries is an important threat to the oral health, well-being, and quality of life of the elderly. The accumulation of the predisposing factors, together with the increasing number of aged people with increasing number of their own teeth, is a growing concern for the clinicians and policy makers alike. But age is not the only factor to consider. For example, patients with removable partial denture or fixed prosthodontic structures, orthodontic appliances or systematic diseases with or without medication may be affected.

Is this book important? Definitely, it is! It is a general assumption that dentin caries is the same whether it occurs in enamel-covered crown or root surface, and the same preventative strategies apply for fissure and root surface caries. I personally do believe this is a false assumption: as a disease, root caries is definitely an entity of its own. The population at risk, risk factors, microbiology, the critical pH for demineralization, the role of endogenous preventive and destructive factors, the progression rate, etc. are significantly different between coronal enamel and root caries [2]. Therefore, our knowledge of the pathogenesis, prevention, and operative treatment of pit-and-fissure or smooth surface enamel caries may not be enough to face the challenge of root caries.

The volume title, as short and simple as it is, tells it all. This monograph takes the reader from the epidemiology of root caries through its biological determinants and lesion assessment and features to build up a comprehensive background for the last part of the book, preventive and operative therapies. This volume has brought together current knowledge and concepts relating to root caries in a comprehensive and lucid fashion. After all, only after understanding the patients at risk and risk factors, and the pathological mechanisms and features of the disease, will the clinician be fully equipped to successfully fight and win the battle. The significance of the text stems from the contributions of distinguished scientists and authorities in this field.

The problem has been recognized, it has been under active research and a lot has been published in dentistry literature, too. Simple PubMed search with key words "root caries" and "review" resulted in over 300 hits. Therefore, it is surprising that even an extensive search for a textbook focusing specifically on root caries failed to find any. This volume of *Monographs in Oral Science* fills this enormous gap, and I am fully confident that it will be welcomed by the under- and postgraduate students, teachers, researchers, and practicing dentists alike.

Enjoy!

Leo Tjäderhane, DDS, PhD, Professor
Department of Oral and Maxillofacial Diseases, University of Helsinki, and Helsinki University Hospital, Helsinki, Finland
Research Unit of Oral Health Sciences, and Medical Research Center Oulu (MRC Oulu), Oulu University Hospital and University of Oulu, Oulu, Finland

References

1 Walls A: Aging – a call to arms! J Dent Res 2017;96:721–722.

2 Takahashi N, Nyvad B: Ecological hypothesis of dentin and root caries. Caries Res 2016;50:422–431.

Carrilho MRO (ed): Root Caries: From Prevalence to Therapy.
Monogr Oral Sci. Basel, Karger, 2017, vol 26, pp 1–8 (DOI: 10.1159/000479301)

Incidence, Prevalence and Global Distribution of Root Caries

Martina Hayes · Francis Burke · Patrick Finbarr Allen

Restorative Dentistry, Cork University Dental School and Hospital, Wilton, Cork, Ireland

Abstract

High quality epidemiological data are essential for both the development of national oral health policies and cost-effective targeting of resources. Unfortunately, a high level of clinical heterogeneity between studies in this area makes it difficult, and inappropriate, to try to produce any definitive figures on the global prevalence or incidence of root caries. Published studies have reported wide ranges for the prevalence of root caries (25–100%) and the mean Root Caries Index (9.7–38.7). The reported range for annual root caries incidence is also wide, from 10.1 to 40.6%. While more research is needed in this area, most studies conclude that the burden of root caries is high in the older age population.

Introduction

Unfortunately, estimating the prevalence and incidence of root caries can be challenging as loss of teeth confounds the data and the diagnostic criteria for root caries differ between studies. In addition to the differences in diagnostic criteria applied to root caries, epidemiological studies of root caries report their findings in a variety of ways using different indices. There was great interest in the epidemiology of root caries among the dental research community in the 1970s and 1980s. During this time, a number of epidemiological studies were published. Many of these simply counted the number of carious and restored root surfaces and presented it as root decayed and filled surfaces (RDFS). Some studies felt that restorations on the root surface could not definitely be attributed to past caries experience and felt it was more accurate to report root decayed surfaces. Others counted the number of teeth which had evidence of root caries or previously restored root caries and presented root decayed and filled teeth.

Sumney et al. [1], in 1973, reported the percentage of the population with one or more root surface caries lesions and also presented the average number of lesions per person per tooth available. In 1980, Banting et al. [2] reported the percentage of the population with at least one filled or decayed root surface and also the mean number of decayed root lesions per patient alongside the mean number of restored root surfaces per patient. As further studies were published during this period, researchers began to highlight the inconsistent reporting methods and the difficulty in comparing the results of studies [3, 4].

In 1980, Katz [5] proposed a new measure which he named the Root Caries Index (RCI) for scoring and reporting root surface caries. From the mid-1980s onwards, the RCI became one of the 2 standard measures used for reporting root caries prevalence (the other being RDFS), with most studies reporting both in conjunction to give as rounded a picture as possible. While there is no doubt that the RCI is imperfect, it has yet to be superseded by a more useful measure. Given the lack of consensus on a definition for root caries and the considerable debate about how best to measure it, it can be seen how complicated the epidemiology of this disease is. Authors writing about root caries have been calling for increased agreement in this area for over forty years [3, 6]. In light of the level of clinical heterogeneity between studies in this area, it is difficult, and inappropriate, to try to produce any definitive figures on the prevalence or incidence of root caries. However, it is interesting to look at the variety of populations in which root caries has been studied and the methods used to collect the data.

Prevalence of Root Caries

Prevalence data from cross-sectional studies serve a number of purposes. These data are used to monitor the amount of disease existing in a population, to delineate the characteristics of people who have the disease, to generate hypotheses regarding the etiology of the disease, and to plan public oral health services. The use of cross-sectional studies to identify the association between risk factors and a disease are limited, however, the fact is that they are carried out at a single time point and give no indication of the sequence of events – whether exposure occurred before, after or during the onset of the disease outcome. This being so, it is impossible to infer causality. As the term "risk factor" implies causality, it may be more accurate to describe any associations as "risk indicators" or "risk markers" for the disease.

Examining epidemiologic studies of root caries reveal numerous threats to their external and internal validities. Very few studies of root caries use a random sampling technique. Most studies recruit volunteers according to pre-defined criteria. These criteria are unique to each study, which impedes cross-study comparisons and limit generalizability. The notable exceptions to this are the national surveys [7, 8]. Studies recruiting volunteers should be interpreted with caution unless they can be proven to be representative or are a subpopulation of interest in their own right, for example, individuals with Alzheimer's disease [9]. Studies on root caries prevalence have been reported for institutionalized elderly [2], independently living elderly [10], those attending day centers [11], adults in fluoridated areas [12], adults in non-fluoridated areas [13], urban dwellers, and rural dwellers [14], as well as the notable Piedmont 65+ studies which looked at African-Americans and Caucasians in North Carolina [15]. Many of the studies reported baseline data from large clinical trials [12, 16, 17]. Clinical trials include selected populations, designed to maximize the likelihood of finding differences between 2 therapies and are often not representative of a general population of interest.

The studies involving some type of sampling frame should provide estimates of prevalence, with proper weighting for the sampling design and unbiased responses. Unfortunately, this level of reporting is rare in root caries epidemiology. An exception to this is the study of Locker et al. [18], which reported a 26% response rate for individuals aged 50 and older. It was not possible to identify any clinical studies which reported the characteristics of non-responders. This is expected as participation in any research is voluntary and it may not be possible to gather any form of data on those who choose not to participate. National surveys, however, should be able to report on the age profile and gender of non-responders as it is assumed that this knowledge would be available prior to random sampling to ensure a representative sample is achieved. A paper was published reporting the findings of the First Uruguayan National Oral Health Survey [19], which indicated a 20% non-response rate among the total population invited to participate. However, further information on the characteristics of non-responders was reported in a separate document which was not available in English [20].

While studies report good inter- and intra-examiner reproducibility, they each diagnose root caries according to different field conditions, on different populations, using differing criteria for root caries. Some studies only refer to untreated root caries when reporting root caries prevalence [21], while others regard treated and untreated root caries equally or present them separately [2]. There is additional complexity when researchers add in descriptors, such as quiescent, active, inactive, or recurrent. It can then be difficult to decipher whether they have included "inactive" lesions in their calculations of RDFS or RCI.

Many of the exposures of interest in root caries epidemiology are specific and reproducible, such as age and gender. However, others such as xerostomia are more likely to vary between studies depending on whether the investigators used a questionnaire to determine self-reported oral dryness [17], or used a quantitative measure such as stimulated saliva collection over a measured time period [22]. Another example is one study which reported that root caries was correlated with decayed-missing-filled-teeth but did not specify if decayed-missing-filled-teeth was calculated from 28 or 32 teeth and whether coronal decay was measured at cavitation level or not [12]. Many studies also investigate the relationship between socioeconomic status and root caries. A recent study categorized participants using Kuppuswamy's classification [23], while many others rely on self-reported income and level of education [11, 22].

As can be seen, there is substantial clinical heterogeneity between studies reporting on root caries prevalence and so it would be misleading to attempt to synthesize this data to produce a global estimate of root caries prevalence. Table 1 briefly describes the settings of some studies reporting on root caries prevalence and Table 2 lists the estimated root caries prevalence to illustrate the wide range reported.

Incidence of Root Caries

For similar reasons outlined above, estimating the true incidence of root caries is extremely challenging and fraught with inconsistencies. Also, there can be confusion when authors refer to incidence and increment. The incidence of root caries refers to the proportion of individuals in who any new root caries is observed over a given time period. Root caries increment refers to the number of root surfaces per person, which develop new root caries over a given period of time.

Longitudinal dental caries studies generally take 2 forms: a cohort study that is observational and attempts to describe, model, or predict new disease; and a clinical trial that is experimental in nature and attempts to report new disease incidence while concurrently testing a new intervention. Clinical trials on interventions for root caries tend to select populations who are at high risk of developing new root caries within a relatively short time, for example, patients who are xerostomic post-radiotherapy to the head and neck regions [24–26]. This is convenient from a research perspective as enough new cases of root caries can be observed to determine if there is any difference between groups within a relatively short period of time. This data is only generalizable to a very specific study population and should not be included in attempts to find the true population incidence for root caries.

Table 1. Studies reporting root caries prevalence (continued over following pages)

Authors	Country	Population	Number of participants	Reported measures
Banting et al. [2]	Canada	Institutionalized adults (mean age 67.9 years)	59	Root caries prevalence
Beck et al. [10]	USA	Independently living adults aged 65+ years	520	Root caries prevalence
Locker et al. [18]	Canada	Independently living adults aged 50+ years (data presented separately for 65+)	138	Root caries prevalence, RDFS, exposed root surfaces
Luan et al. [45]	China	Urban and rural adults aged 20–80 years (data presented separately for 60+)	544 (238 M, 306 F)	Root caries prevalence, exposed root surfaces
Fejerskov et al. [46]	Denmark	Independently living adults aged 60–80 years	90 (46 M, 44 F)	Sound root surfaces, Active and inactive root surface caries, RCI
Papas et al. [47]	USA	Adults aged 40+ years (data presented separately for 65+)	180 (61 M, 119 F)	RDFS
Slade and Spencer [48]	Australia	Non-institutionalized aged 60+	853 (497 M, 356 F)	RDFS, exposed root surfaces, RCI
Närhi et al. [49]	Finland	Dentate elderly (mean age 79.3 years)	196 (56 M, 127 F)	RDFS, exposed root surfaces
Splieth et al. [50]	Germany	Adults aged 20–79 years (data presented separately for 65+)	982 (545 M, 437 F)	RDFS, exposed root surfaces, RCI
Kularatne and Ekanayake [51]	Sri Lanka	Urban dwellers aged 60+ years	600 (281 M, 319 F)	RDFS, exposed root surfaces, RCI
Islas-Granillo et al. [52]	Mexico	Institutionalized and non-institutionalized aged 60+ years	85 (25 M, 60 F)	Exposed root surfaces, RCI
Ellefsen et al. [9]	Denmark	Older adults with Alzheimer's disease	61 (22 M, 39 F)	Root caries prevalence, RDFS
Mamai-Homata et al. [11]	Greece	Older adults in day centers aged 65+ years	749 (427 M, 322 F)	Root caries prevalence, RDFS, RCI
Chi et al. [22]	USA	Adult dental attenders aged 45+ years (data presented separately for 65+)	368 (204 M, 164 F)	Root caries prevalence
Silva et al. [33]	Australia	Institutionalized adults (mean age 83 years)	243 (80 M, 163 F)	Root caries, prevalence, RDFS, RCI
Christensen et al. [53]	Denmark	Adults aged 21–89 years (data presented separately for aged 65+)	1,063 aged 65+	Root caries prevalence

Random sampling is preferred when estimating the incidence of any disease as it provides a group from which to generalize the results or conclusions of the study. Quite often, however, random sampling is not practical due to the cost and time constraints. Also, in a disease such as root caries, which is more prevalent in older age groups, it can be logical to focus resources on the population of interest. For example, the most recent oral health survey in Ireland examined 1,196 people aged between 16 and 24 years of age. The mean number of ex-

Table 2. Reported root caries prevalence across studies (nr = not reported)

Study	Prevalence of root caries experience, %	Mean RDFS	Mean RCI
Banting et al. [2], 1980	83	nr	nr
Beck et al. [10], 1985	63	nr	nr
Locker et al. [18], 1989	57	2.6	10.2
Luan et al. [45], 1989	66	nr	nr
Fejerskov et al. [46], 1991	100	7.4	nr
Papas et al. [47], 1992	nr	5.6	nr
Slade and Spencer [48], 1997	nr	3.1	11.9
Närhi et al. [49], 1997	37	5.2	nr
Splieth et al. [50], 2004	53	8.6	10.3
Kularatne and Ekanayake [51], 2007	90	3.8	25.0
Islas-Granillo et al. [52], 2012	96	nr	37.7
Ellefsen et al. [9], 2012	75	10.3	ns
Mamai-Homata et al. [11], 2012	38	2.7	9.7
Chi et al. [22], 2013	25	nr	nr
Silva et al. [33], 2013	77	6.5	38.7
Christensen et al. [53], 2015	45	nr	nr

posed roots was 1.2 and the mean root decayed and filled teeth was 0 [7]. From the point of view of a governmental agency or funding body, it would not be justifiable to spend limited resources to determine the incidence of root caries in this population. The sample size should be large and the follow-up longer, and it would be difficult to see the benefit of this data for a wider society.

As root caries is a disease seen predominantly in older adults, it is justifiable to limit a study population to this group. Unfortunately, this group is not easily defined. Most developed countries have accepted the chronological age of 65 years as a definition of 'elderly' or older person. While this definition is somewhat arbitrary, it is associated with the age at which one can begin to receive pension benefits. Although there are commonly used definitions of old age (such as 65 years and older), there is no general agreement on the age at which a person becomes old. The common use of a calendar age to mark the threshold of old age assumes equivalence with biological age, yet at the same time, it is generally accepted that these 2 are not necessarily synonymous. Older adults can be subdivided into the 3rd age and the 4th age [27], or the young-old, old-old, and oldest-old [28, 29]. They can also be categorized according to frailty using a measure, such as the Canadian Study of Health and Ageing frailty scores [30]. This system of categorization was advocated in the Seattle Care Pathway for securing oral health in older patients [31].

Frail or institutionalized older adults have a higher prevalence of root caries than other older populations, and so it may be clinically useful to study the root caries incidence of this population separately compared to that among independently living older adults [32, 33]. However, caution should be exercised with definitions in this area; many authors use the terms frail and dependent to describe those in nursing homes, yet one study specifically recruited non-frail individuals living in nursing homes [34]. This indicates that living in a nursing home is not synonymous with frailty. And so it can be difficult to examine the literature and separate out data for frail older adults and non-frail older adults.

The diagnosis of root caries is a matter of considerable debate, and one study may record a new lesion as one which can be probed with a sharp explorer [35] while another might not consider it as a lesion in their estimation of root caries incidence. Some studies calculated RCI by including both active and inactive lesions as root caries while another study treated inactive lesions as sound-exposed root surfaces in statistical calculations [36]. Another issue arose when calculating root caries increment; that is the classification of new lesions associated with an existing restoration (i.e., recurrent caries). While this is a new caries activity, it can go unrecorded if the authors calculate root caries incidence by subtracting the baseline RDFS from the RDFS at follow-up [37, 38]. In some cases, it can be impossible to determine how recurrent caries were interpreted in the calculation of root caries incidence [39]. To add to the heterogeneity, adjustments for "reversals" (changes from filled or decayed root surfaces to sound) are made by some researchers [40] but not by others [39].

The findings of 6 studies conducted among populations living in "advanced market economies" were summarized in one systematic review and a meta-analysis of root caries incidence performed [41]. Despite this being a systematic review, there is no published search strategy, either in the article itself or in the supplementary material. It is consequentially impossible to attempt to replicate the systematic review or for another researcher to update it in the future.

It can be determined from the article that studies published before 1980 were excluded, and so were the research not published in English. Populations such as institutionalized adults, xerostomic individuals, and those exposed to caries-prevention measures other than fluoride toothpaste and fluoridation were excluded. Interestingly, studies which did not provide evidence that informed consent had been obtained from subjects and/or approval obtained from an Internal Review Board were excluded. However, it was not stated which studies were excluded for these reasons and whether inclusion of these studies would significantly affect the estimated summary root caries increment. Only studies which reported variance, standard deviation or standard error of their estimated increment or attack rate were included. Where possible, the authors reported estimates of new disease that did not subtract out the "reversals" in an effort to make the findings of studies, which adjusted for negative reversals, more comparable with studies which did not.

Eleven studies were identified for inclusion in the review. The summary annual root caries incidence for 9 studies was 23.7% (95% CI 17.1–30.2). Two of the included studies did not report this measure. The range in individual studies went from 10.1% in Canada [42] to 40.6% in Washington DC, USA [43]. Five of the 11 studies had estimated annual root caries attack rate (i.e., number of surfaces decayed per 100 surfaces at risk). This figure ranged from 0.9% in Sweden [44] to 3.9% in Washington DC, USA [43]. The summary annual root caries attack rate was 1.9% (95% CI 0.9–2.8). The authors do advise caution when interpreting this summary root caries incidence due to the level of heterogeneity present. While there are limitations to this systematic review, it does appear to have some generalizability to first world economies and could serve as a comparison for future longitudinal studies.

Conclusions

Due to the high level of heterogeneity between studies, it is not possible to estimate the global prevalence or incidence of root caries. Future studies which are integrated into large longitudinal studies on aging are likely to provide valuable data with greater generalizability. However, a consensus on the definition of a root caries lesion is needed to allow for future meta-synthesis of studies.

References

1 Sumney DL, Jordan HV, Englander HR: The prevalence of root surface caries in selected populations. J Periodontol 1973; 44:500–504.

2 Banting DW, Ellen RP, Fillery ED: Prevalence of root surface caries among institutionalized older persons. Community Dent Oral Epidemiol 1980;8:84–88.

3 Hazen SP, Chilton NW, Mumma RD Jr: The problem of root caries. I. Literature review and clinical description. J Am Dent Assoc 1973;86:137–144.

4 Banting DW: Epidemiology of root caries. Gerodontology 1986;5:5–11.

5 Katz RV: Assessing root caries in populations: the evolution of the root caries index. J Public Health Dent 1980;40: 7–16.

6 Ritter AV, Shugars DA, Bader JD: Root caries risk indicators: a systematic review of risk models. Community Dent Oral Epidemiol 2010;38:383–397.

7 Whelton H, Crowley E, O'Mullane D, et al: Oral Health of Irish Adults 2000–2002. Department of Health, Dublin, Ireland, 2007.

8 Kim JK, Baker LA, Seirawan H, Crimmins EM: Prevalence of oral health problems in U.S. adults, NHANES 1999–2004: exploring differences by age, education, and race/ethnicity. Spec Care Dentist 2012;32:234–241.

9 Ellefsen BS, Morse DE, Waldemar G, Holm-Pedersen P: Indicators for root caries in Danish persons with recently diagnosed Alzheimer's disease. Gerodontology 2012;29:194–202.

10 Beck JD, Hunt RJ, Hand JS, Field HM: Prevalence of root and coronal caries in a noninstitutionalized older population. J Am Dent Assoc 1985;111:964–967.

11 Mamai-Homata E, Topitsoglou V, Oulis C, Margaritis V, Polychronopoulou A: Risk indicators of coronal and root caries in Greek middle aged adults and senior citizens. BMC Public Health 2012; 12:484.

12 Burt BA, Ismail AI, Eklund S: Root caries in an optimally fluoridated and a high-fluoride community. J Dent Res 1986;65:1154–1158.

13 Stamm JV, Banting DW: Comparison of root caries prevalence in adults with life-long residence in fluoridated and non-fluoridated communities. J Dent Res 1980;59:405–410.

14 Du M, Jiang H, Tai B, Zhou Y, Wu B, Bian Z: Root caries patterns and risk factors of middle-aged and elderly people in China. Community Dent Oral Epidemiol 2009;37:260–266.

15 Graves RC, Beck JD, Disney JA, Drake CW: Root caries prevalence in black and white North Carolina adults over age 65. J Public Health Dent 1992;52:94–101.

16 Jensen ME, Kohout F: The effect of a fluoridated dentifrice on root and coronal caries in an older adult population. J Am Dent Assoc 1988;117:829–832.

17 Ritter AV, Preisser JS, Chung Y, et al: Risk indicators for the presence and extent of root caries among caries-active adults enrolled in the Xylitol for Adult Caries Trial (X-ACT). Clin Oral Investig 2012;16:1647–1657.

18 Locker D, Slade GD, Leake JL: Prevalence of and factors associated with root decay in older adults in Canada. J Dent Res 1989;68:768–772.

19 Álvarez L, Liberman J, Abreu S, et al: Dental caries in Uruguayan adults and elders: findings from the first Uruguayan National Oral Health Survey. Cad Saude Publica 2015;31:1663–1672.

20 Lorenzo S, Álvarez R, Blanco S, Peres M: Primer Relevamiento Nacional de Salud Bucal en población joven y adulta uruguaya: aspectos metodológicos. Odontoestomatología 2013;15:8–25.

21 Lohse W, Carter H, Brunelle J: The prevalence of root surface caries in a military population. Military Med 1977;142:700–703.

22 Chi DL, Berg JH, Kim AS, Scott J: Correlates of root caries experience in middle-aged and older adults in the Northwest Practice-based REsearch Collaborative in Evidence-based DENTistry research network. J Am Dent Assoc 2013;144: 507–516.

23 Zhang Q, Jing Q, Gerritsen AE, Witter DJ, Bronkhorst EM, Creugers NH: Dental status of an institutionalized elderly population of 60 years and over in Qingdao, China. Clin Oral Investig 2016;20: 1021–1028.

24 Wood RE, Maxymiw WG, McComb D: A clinical comparison of glass ionomer (polyalkenoate) and silver amalgam restorations in the treatment of Class 5 caries in xerostomic head and neck cancer patients. Oper Dent 1993;18:94–102.

25 McComb D, Erickson RL, Maxymiw WG, Wood RE: A clinical comparison of glass ionomer, resin-modified glass ionomer and resin composite restorations in the treatment of cervical caries in xerostomic head and neck radiation patients. Oper Dent 2002;27:430–437.

26 De Moor RJ, Stassen IG, van 't Veldt Y, Torbeyns D, Hommez GM: Two-year clinical performance of glass ionomer and resin composite restorations in xerostomic head- and neck-irradiated cancer patients. Clin Oral Investig 2011;15: 31–38.

27 Baltes PB, Smith J: New frontiers in the future of aging: from successful aging of the young old to the dilemmas of the fourth age. Gerontology 2003;49:123–135.

28 Smith J, Borchelt M, Maier H, Jopp D: Health and well-being in the young old and oldest old. J Soc Issues 2002;58: 715–732.

29 Chou KL, Chi I: Successful aging among the young-old, old-old, and oldest-old Chinese. Int J Aging Hum Dev 2002;54: 1–14.

30 Rockwood K, Song X, MacKnight C, et al: A global clinical measure of fitness and frailty in elderly people. CMAJ 2005; 173:489–495.

31 Pretty IA, Ellwood RP, Lo EC, et al: The Seattle Care Pathway for securing oral health in older patients. Gerodontology 2014;31:77–87.

32 Baca P, Clavero J, Baca AP, González-Rodríguez MP, Bravo M, Valderrama MJ: Effect of chlorhexidine-thymol varnish on root caries in a geriatric population: a randomized double-blind clinical trial. J Dent 2009;37:679–685.

33 Silva M, Hopcraft M, Morgan M: Dental caries in Victorian nursing homes. Aust Dent J 2014;59:321–328.

34 Tan HP, Lo EC, Dyson JE, Luo Y, Corbet EF: A randomized trial on root caries prevention in elders. J Dent Res 2010;89: 1086–1090.

35 Hahn P, Reinhardt D, Schaller HG, Hellwig E: Root lesions in a group of 50–60 year-old Germans related to clinical and social factors. Clin Oral Investig 1999;3: 168–174.

36 Imazato S, Ikebe K, Nokubi T, Ebisu S, Walls AW: Prevalence of root caries in a selected population of older adults in Japan. J Oral Rehabil 2006;33:137–143.

37 Scheinin A, Pienihäkkinen K, Tiekso J, Holmberg S, Fukuda M, Suzuki A: Multifactorial modeling for root caries prediction: 3-year follow-up results. Community Dent Oral Epidemiol 1994;22:126–129.

38 Sánchez-García S, Reyes-Morales H, Juárez-Cedillo T, Espinel-Bermúdez C, Solórzano-Santos F, García-Peña C: A prediction model for root caries in an elderly population. Community Dent Oral Epidemiol 2011;39:44–52.

39 Powell LV, Leroux BG, Persson RE, Kiyak HA: Factors associated with caries incidence in an elderly population. Community Dent Oral Epidemiol 1998;26:170–176.

40 Gilbert GH, Duncan RP, Dolan TA, Foerster U: Twenty-four month incidence of root caries among a diverse group of adults. Caries Res 2001;35:366–375.

41 Griffin SO, Griffin PM, Swann JL, Zlobin N: Estimating rates of new root caries in older adults. J Dent Res 2004;83:634–638.

42 Locker D, Leake JL: Coronal and root decay experience in older adults in Ontario, Canada. J Public Health Dent 1993;53:158–164.

43 Powell LV, Persson RE, Kiyak HA, Hujoel PP: Caries prevention in a community-dwelling older population. Caries Res 1999;33:333–339.

44 Fure S: Five-year incidence of coronal and root caries in 60-, 70- and 80-year-old Swedish individuals. Caries Res 1997;31:249–258.

45 Luan WM, Baelum V, Chen X, Fejerskov O: Dental caries in adult and elderly Chinese. J Dent Res 1989;68:1771–1776.

46 Fejerskov O, Luan WM, Nyvad B, Budtz-Jørgensen E, Holm-Pedersen P: Active and inactive root surface caries lesions in a selected group of 60- to 80-year-old Danes. Caries Res 1991;25:385–391.

47 Papas A, Joshi A, Giunta J: Prevalence and intraoral distribution of coronal and root caries in middle-aged and older adults. Caries Res 1992;26:459–465.

48 Slade GD, Spencer AJ: Distribution of coronal and root caries experience among persons aged 60+ in South Australia. Aust Dent J 1997;42:178–184.

49 Närhi TO, Vehkalahti MM, Siukosaari P, Ainamo A: Salivary findings, daily medication and root caries in the old elderly. Caries Res 1997;32:5–9.

50 Splieth Ch, Schwahn Ch, Bernhardt O, John U: Prevalence and distribution of root caries in Pomerania, North-East Germany. Caries Res 2004;38:333–340.

51 Kularatne S, Ekanayake L: Root surface caries in older individuals from Sri Lanka. Caries Res 2007;41:252–256.

52 Islas-Granillo H, Borges-Yañez SA, Medina-Solís CE, Casanova-Rosado AJ, Minaya-Sánchez M, Villalobos Rodelo JJ, Maupomé G: Socioeconomic, sociodemographic, and clinical variables associated with root caries in a group of persons age 60 years and older in Mexico. Geriatr Gerontol Int 2012;12:271–276.

53 Christensen LB, Bardow A, Ekstrand K, Fiehn NE, Heitmann BL, Qvist V, Twetman S: Root caries, root surface restorations and lifestyle factors in adult Danes. Acta Odontol Scand 2015;73:467–473.

Martina Hayes
Restorative Dentistry, Cork University Dental School and Hospital
University College Cork
Wilton, Cork T12 E8YV (Ireland)
E-Mail Martina.Hayes@ucc.ie

Carrilho MRO (ed): Root Caries: From Prevalence to Therapy.
Monogr Oral Sci. Basel, Karger, 2017, vol 26, pp 9–14 (DOI: 10.1159/000479302)

Etiology, Risk Factors and Groups of Risk

Martina Hayes · Francis Burke · Patrick Finbarr Allen
Restorative Dentistry, Cork University Dental School and Hospital, Wilton, Cork, Ireland

Abstract
Population aging and the concomitant reduction in tooth loss will have a profound effect on dentistry. In particular, an increase in the prevalence of root caries can be expected. Root caries is not evenly distributed across the population and identification of high-risk groups or individuals would facilitate targeted prevention strategies. Unfortunately, the lack of consensus in the literature on the diagnosis and measurement of root caries makes comparison of studies extremely challenging. At present, we do not have an adequately validated risk assessment tool for root caries. Future research should focus resources on investigating risk indicators, which have been found to be significant in past studies and on externally validating previously described risk models.

Introduction

In many industrialized countries, as birth rates fall and life expectancy increases, the proportion of older adults within the general population is increasing. This trend is predicted to continue at a pace in the 21st century [1]. While the prevalence of chronic medical conditions is high in this cohort, large longitudinal population studies on aging have shown that an increasing number of older adults are independently living, mobile, and active in their communities [2–4]. With increasing numbers of patients retaining natural teeth into old age, the challenge of providing oral healthcare for the aging population is undoubtedly going to increase. An increase in exposed root surfaces in the over 65 age group predisposes this group to a higher prevalence of root caries than younger populations [5].

Root caries is a multi-factorial, bacterially mediated process that results in the destruction of mineralized tooth tissues. Sumney et al. [6] defined root caries as "a cavitation below the cemento-enamel junction, not usually including the adjacent enamel, usually discolored, softened, ill-defined, and involving both cementum and underlying dentine." However, there is no consensus in the literature on the definition of root caries. Disagreement arises over whether or not it includes adjacent enamel, and if so, what proportion of the lesion must be on the root surface [7, 8]. The lack of well-defined terminology in the study of root caries leads to challenges in interpreting the reported prevalence and incidence of root caries.

The root surface may be more vulnerable to mechanical destruction than the crown because the structure and chemical composition of cementum and dentine differ. In a population who are frequently exposed to scaling by dental health professionals, the cementum layer is frequently abraded away, exposing the dentine. Root cementum and dentine are structurally different from enamel and react differently to cariogenic challenges – in particular, the critical pH of dentine and cementum is approximately 6.4 [9] while that of enamel is 5.5 [10].

Schüpbach et al. [11] classified root caries into 3 main categories, based on histopathological features: lesions in cementum, initial lesions in dentine, and advanced lesions in dentine. Microstructural observations of initial root caries lesions reported an outer layer with dentinal tubules partly occluded by peritubular and intratubular dentine deposition and an underlying layer of translucent dentine. Dentinal tubules appear to be sclerosed by precipitation of calcium and phosphate ions and contain "ghosts" of bacteria and fine-granular crystals. Stagnating or quiescent lesions are characterized by a surface layer which has a high mineral content, and viable bacteria are absent from the dentinal tubules [12]. Conversely, in progressing active lesions, the superficial layer displays diffuse bacterial penetration, and an intermediate area of demineralizing dentine can be seen above the translucent zone of dentine [11].

The etiology of the initiation and progression of root caries is the combination of cariogenic bacteria and fermentable carbohydrate on the root surface [13]. *Lactobacillus, Streptococcus mutans,* and *Actinomyces* have been implicated in the development of root caries [14, 15]. However, not all studies which have examined these microorganisms have found a significant correlation between their levels in saliva and root caries [16]. Modern sequencing techniques studying the human microbiome are likely to bring further understanding of the microbial pathogenesis of root caries in the near future [17].

Risk Factors Associated with Root Caries

As root caries is not randomly distributed within the population, many researchers have attempted to identify factors which may predispose an individual to the disease. Root caries is a preventable disease; however, access to care, compliance issues, and cost may preclude the use of a preventive intervention on the entire population. It is known that one-third of the older adult population bears most of the root caries burden [18–20]. Therefore, if these individuals could be identified prior to developing the disease, targeted prevention measures could be delivered. A variety of risk indicators have been associated with root caries in cross-sectional and longitudinal studies but the heterogeneous results of these studies are difficult to interpret. This is primarily due to the lack of consensus on the definition and diagnostic criteria for root caries. Additionally, cause-effect relationships cannot be established from associations based on cross-sectional studies [21].

Studies on risk factors for root caries have been conducted in a number of countries including Finland, the United States, Australia, Mexico, and Japan [22–26]. Recruited sample populations have included low income older people [27], adults under the age of 65 years [27], adults with dementia [24], and HIV-seropositive women [28]. Root caries is a complex, multifactorial disease and it is not clear whether the risk factors for this disease are the same across diverse populations.

A systematic review of root caries risk indicators from published predictive risk models was conducted by researchers in the University of North Carolina [16]. It included English articles published between 1970 and June 2009 reporting longitudinal root caries data. The search strategy is well described and there is a flowchart summary of the search process, including reasons for excluding articles. An online appendix with listed excluded articles and their reason for exclusion was also provided for readers.

Thirteen articles were selected for inclusion in the review. The follow-up time of the studies ranged from one to 10 years (median 3 years). The sample sizes ranged from 23 participants to 723 (mean 264, SD 203). The authors assessed the overall quality of the studies as moderate, but felt that the quality of the statistical modeling approach was poor. Ninety-five variables were examined across 13 studies. The most commonly tested variable was root decayed and filled surfaces (RDFS) at baseline, which had been tested in 12 of the 13 studies. This was found to be significant in 7 out of the 12 studies. The second most frequently examined variable was age, which was included in 10 studies and was significant in 2 [28, 29].

Smoking was included as a variable in 9 studies but was only significant in one of these [28]. Medication use was found to be significant in 2 out of 9 studies [30, 31]. Gender was a significant variable in 2 out of 8 studies [24, 32], with males having an increased risk compared to females. Five out of 7 studies found a significant association between the number of teeth at baseline (or its inverse, missing teeth) and root caries incidence [23, 28, 31, 33, 34].

Table 1 presents a summary of the variables examined in more than one study. It is difficult to come to any conclusion about the role of variables which have been examined even across many studies as each study may define the variable in their own way. Taking the variable "number of teeth at baseline" as an example; some studies use this as a continuous variable in their analysis [28, 31]. While another study subdivided the number of teeth at baseline into 4 categories and reported that those that had between 9 and 16 teeth at baseline were at an increased risk of caries compared to groups that had both more and less teeth [23]. To add to the complexity, association directionality was not the same across all studies which found this variable to be significant.

Table 1. Summary of variables tested as potential risk indicators for root caries. Adapted from Ritter et al. [16]

Variable	Times tested	Times significant
Baseline RDFS	12	7
Age	10	2
Smoking	9	1
Medication use	9	2
Gender	8	2
Lactobacilli counts	8	3
Streptococcus mutans counts	8	1
Saliva flow rate	8	1
Number of teeth at baseline	7	5
Saliva buffer capacity	6	1
Diet	6	0
Dental visit pattern	5	1
Plaque index	4	3
Baseline coronal DFS	4	0
Education	4	0
Oral hygiene status	3	0
Ethnicity	3	1
Prosthetic crown/FPD	3	1
Use of interdental cleaning aid	3	1
Attachment loss	3	1
Use of removable partial denture	2	2
Candida	2	1
BMI	2	0
Marital status	2	0
Alcohol use	2	0
Income	2	0

Another example is the variable "medications." One study looked at the relationship between the number of medications taken per day and root caries incidence [31], another at the number of medications taken which have a known side effect of xerostomia [27], and yet another at antihistamines alone [30].

The systematic review concluded that there is substantial variation among root caries risk indicator studies relative to variable selection, sample size, outcomes, assessment methods, incidence periods, association directionality, and analysis techniques. These factors limit the applicability of the findings to guide targeted root caries prevention strategies. Future studies are needed and should emphasize variables which have been frequently tested and found to be significant in more than one study [16].

A literature search beyond the date of this systematic review identified 2 longitudinal studies reporting risk models [25, 26]. The first of these studies examined the relationship between 31 variables and root caries increment in a 12-months period in 531 elderly Mexican participants [25]. The final prediction model included 6 risk factors for root caries: limitations in basic daily living activities, smoking, not using dental mouthwash, high Streptococcus mutans count, ≥6 healthy root surfaces at baseline, and a baseline root caries index of 8% or higher.

The other longitudinal study was conducted in Japan on participants aged between 20 and 59 years [26]. One hundred and eighteen men and 23 women participated in this study on coronal and root caries. They reported the 5-year root caries incidence in individuals within this cohort who were at risk of root caries, that is, who had some gingival recession. It was not reported how many participants were included in the root caries data analysis. It was found that the risk of root caries increased with: age, the presence of any gingival recession, having at least one filled or decayed root surface at baseline, and having at least 5 filled or decayed coronal tooth surfaces at baseline.

Prediction Modeling for Root Caries

The final result of many cross-sectional studies and longitudinal studies are prediction models, usually generated using some form of logistic regression. Multifactorial modeling has attempted to show the interrelations and interactions of risk indicators with the occurrence of the disease. Some authors have advocated that a successful model should include one or more social, behavioral, microbiologic, environmental or clinical variables [35]. Modeling is typically based on a dichotomized dependent variable, usually no versus some root caries increment over time.

It is necessary to evaluate the power of a predictive model to determine if it can be used for screenings at a public health level. To be useful, a working caries prediction model should produce a sensitivity of 0.75 or higher and a specificity level of at least 0.85 [36]. Another cut-off suggested for a good diagnostic test is a combined sensitivity and specificity of at least 160% [37]. A high specificity ensures that the healthcare system would not be over burdened by too many false positives, which would result in the overtreatment of individuals with preventive approaches and, therefore, the overuse of limited resources [38].

An important limitation of the models reported in the literature to date is their lack of independent validation. Before considering whether to use a clinical prediction model, it is essential that its predictive performance be empirically evaluated in datasets that were not used to develop the model [39]. Only one paper in the root caries literature reported an attempt to internally validate the model on a sub-sample of patients [32].

Of the 15 published root caries risk models, 10 include past root caries experience in some form (i.e., RDFS, Root Caries Index [RCI], RCI_{log}) as a significant predictive variable. This finding compromises the use of these models as true preventive tools as they rely on past disease experience to predict future experience, thereby limiting the ability to identify a high risk individual before they become exposed to the disease. None of the 5 studies which did not include past root caries experience in their predictive model report the sensitivity and specificity of their model [24, 27, 28, 30, 31]. Three of the studies do not provide any summary statistic of the predictive power of their models [27, 28, 30]. The remaining 2 studies report pseudo R^2 statistics. Chalmers et al. [24] reported an R^2 of 0.075 and Fure [31] reported an R^2 of 0.36. Given that an R^2 value of <0.5 indicates poor predictive value [40], neither of the predictive models from these studies are likely to be clinically useful.

The model reported by Scheinin et al. [22] had a sensitivity of 77.6% and a specificity of 76.6%. This results in a Youden's index of 0.54; the highest of the root caries prediction models identified in the literature. Youden's *J* statistic (also called Youden's index) is a single statistic that captures the performance of a dichotomous diagnostic test. It is calculated as follows:

$$J = \text{sensitivity} + \text{specificity} - 1$$

This model included 3 variables: past root caries experience (RDFS), Candida, and Lactobacilli levels. This model does not reach the minimum criteria set out in the literature of a combined sensitivity and specificity of 160%. It is the most promising model to date but would need external validation to confirm the reproducibility of these reported sensitivity and specificity levels in a different population.

The Cariogram is an interactive computer-based caries risk assessment program which was developed in Malmö, Sweden, by Bratthall and Hänsel Petersson [41]. The validity of the Cariogram for root caries prediction among adults (55–75 years old) has been explored [19]. The authors reported that subjects assigned to the highest risk group by the computer program developed more root caries (mean 2.05 surfaces) compared to those in the lowest risk group (0.26 surfaces). No outcomes related to the sensitivity and specificity for coronal or root caries predictions were explored. A systematic review rated the quality of this study as poor as there was no attempt to control the confounding factors and there was no reported measure of examiner reliability [42].

Conclusions

There is a lack of consensus around the diagnostic criteria for root caries and this impedes cross study comparisons and meta-synthesis of available data. To date, there is no adequately validated risk assessment tool for root caries which meets the accepted sensitivity and specificity thresholds for a good diagnostic test. While many studies have published prediction models for root caries, there is a need for external validation of any future models which show promise in root caries prediction. Future models should also aim to include variables other than past root caries experience. Inclusion of past root caries experience compromises the use of these models as true preventive tools as they preclude the opportunity to identify a high risk individual before they become exposed to the disease.

References

1 WHO: Active Ageing: A Policy Framework: A Contribution of the World Health Organization to the Second United Nations World Assembly on Ageing. Madrid, WHO, 2002.

2 Sonnega A, Faul JD, Ofstedal MB, Langa KM, Phillips JW, Weir DR: Cohort profile: the Health and Retirement Study (HRS). Int J Epidemiol 2014;43:576–585.

3 Banks J, Nazroo J, Steptoe A: The Dynamics of Ageing: Evidence from the English Longitudinal Study of Ageing 2002–10 (Wave 5), 2012.

4 Murphy C: Demographic and Health Profile of Older Adults Utilising Public Health Nursing Services in Ireland: Findings from the Irish Longitudinal Study on Ageing (TILDA), 2015.

5 Kelly M, Steele J, Nuttall N, et al: Adult Dental Health Survey – Oral Health in the United Kingdom 1998. London, The Stationery Office, 2000.

6 Sumney DL, Jordan HV, Englander HR: The prevalence of root surface caries in selected populations. J Periodontol 1973; 44:500–504.

7 Banting DW, Ellen RP, Fillery ED: Prevalence of root surface caries among institutionalized older persons. Community Dent Oral Epidemiol 1980;8:84–88.

8 Katz RV, Hazen SP, Chilton NW, Mumma RD Jr: Prevalence and intraoral distribution of root caries in an adult population. Caries Res 1982;16:265–271.
9 Melberg JR: Demineralization and remineralization of root surface caries. Gerodontology 1986;5:25–31.
10 Stephan RM, Miller BF: A quantitative method for evaluating physical and chemical agents which modify production of acids in bacterial plaques on human teeth. J Dent Res 1943;22:45–51.
11 Schüpbach P, Guggenheim B, Lutz F: Histopathology of root surface caries. J Dent Res 1990;69:1195–1204.
12 Schüpbach P, Lutz F, Guggenheim B: Human root caries: histopathology of arrested lesions. Caries Res 1992;26: 153–164.
13 Clarkson JE: Epidemiology of root caries. Am J Dent 1995;8:329–334.
14 Beighton D, Lynch E: Comparison of selected microflora of plaque and underlying carious dentine associated with primary root caries lesions. Caries Res 1995;29:154–158.
15 Brailsford SR, Lynch E, Beighton D: The isolation of Actinomyces naeslundii from sound root surfaces and root carious lesions. Caries Res 1998;32:100–106.
16 Ritter AV, Shugars DA, Bader JD: Root caries risk indicators: a systematic review of risk models. Community Dent Oral Epidemiol 2010;38:383–397.
17 Chen L, Qin B, Du M, et al: Extensive description and comparison of human supra-gingival microbiome in root caries and health. PLoS One 2015; 10:e0117064.
18 Anusavice KJ: Preservative dentistry: the standard of care for the 21st century. J Public Health Dent 1995;55:67–68.
19 Hänsel Petersson G, Fure S, Bratthall D: Evaluation of a computer-based caries risk assessment program in an elderly group of individuals. Acta Odontol Scand 2003;61:164–171.
20 Griffin SO, Griffin PM, Swann JL, Zlobin N: Estimating rates of new root caries in older adults. J Dent Res 2004;83:634–638.
21 Levin KA: Study design III: cross-sectional studies. Evid Based Dent 2006;7: 24–25.
22 Scheinin A, Pienihäkkinen K, Tiekso J, Holmberg S, Fukuda M, Suzuki A: Multifactorial modeling for root caries prediction: 3-year follow-up results. Community Dent Oral Epidemiol 1994;22: 126–129.
23 Gilbert GH, Duncan RP, Dolan TA, Foerster U: Twenty-four month incidence of root caries among a diverse group of adults. Caries Res 2001;35: 366–375.
24 Chalmers JM, Carter KD, Spencer AJ: Caries incidence and increments in community-living older adults with and without dementia. Gerodontology 2002; 19:80–94.
25 Sánchez-García S, Reyes-Morales H, Juárez-Cedillo T, Espinel-Bermúdez C, Solórzano-Santos F, García-Peña C: A prediction model for root caries in an elderly population. Community Dent Oral Epidemiol 2011;39:44–52.
26 Sugihara N, Maki Y, Kurokawa A, Matsukubo T: Cohort study on incidence of coronal and root caries in Japanese adults. Bull Tokyo Dent Coll 2014;55: 125–130.
27 Powell LV, Leroux BG, Persson RE, Kiyak HA: Factors associated with caries incidence in an elderly population. Community Dent Oral Epidemiol 1998; 26:170–176.
28 Phelan JA, Mulligan R, Nelson E, et al: Dental caries in HIV-seropositive women. J Dent Res 2004;83:869–873.
29 Locker D: Incidence of root caries in an older Canadian population. Community Dent Oral Epidemiol 1996;24:403–407.
30 Lawrence HP, Hunt RJ, Beck JD: Three-year root caries incidence and risk modeling in older adults in North Carolina. J Public Health Dent 1995;55:69–78.
31 Fure S: Ten-year cross-sectional and incidence study of coronal and root caries and some related factors in elderly Swedish individuals. Gerodontology 2004;21:130–140.
32 Powell LV, Mancl LA, Senft GD: Exploration of prediction models for caries risk assessment of the geriatric population. Community Dent Oral Epidemiol 1991;19:291–295.
33 Ravald N, Birkhed D: Prediction of root caries in periodontally treated patients maintained with different fluoride programmes. Caries Res 1992;26:450–458.
34 Joshi A, Papas AS, Giunta J: Root caries incidence and associated risk factors in middle-aged and older adults. Gerodontology 1993;10:83–89.
35 Banting DW: Epidemiology of root caries. Gerodontology 1986;5:5–11.
36 Stamm JW, Disney JA, Graves RC, Bohannan HM, Abernathy JR: The University of North Carolina caries risk assessment study. I: rationale and content. J Public Health Dent 1988;48:225–232.
37 Kingman A, Little W, Gomez I, et al: Salivary levels of Streptococcus mutans and lactobacilli and dental caries experiences in a US adolescent population. Community Dent Oral Epidemiol 1988; 16:98–103.
38 Zero D, Fontana M, Lennon AM: Clinical applications and outcomes of using indicators of risk in caries management. J Dent Educ 2001;65:1126–1132.
39 Steyerberg EW, Moons KG, van der Windt DA, et al: Prognosis Research Strategy (PROGRESS) 3: prognostic model research. PLoS Med 2013; 10:e1001381.
40 Hosmer DW Jr, Lemeshow S, Sturdivant RX: Applied Logistic Regression. John Wiley & Sons, 2013.
41 Bratthall D, Hänsel Petersson G: Cariogram – a multifactorial risk assessment model for a multifactorial disease. Community Dent Oral Epidemiol 2005;33: 256–264.
42 Tellez M, Gomez J, Pretty I, Ellwood R, Ismail A: Evidence on existing caries risk assessment systems: are they predictive of future caries? Community Dent Oral Epidemiol 2013;41:67–78.

Martina Hayes
Restorative Dentistry, Cork University Dental School and Hospital
University College Cork
Wilton, Cork T12 E8YV (Ireland)
E-Mail Martina.Hayes@ucc.ie

Carrilho MRO (ed): Root Caries: From Prevalence to Therapy.
Monogr Oral Sci. Basel, Karger, 2017, vol 26, pp 15–25 (DOI: 10.1159/000479303)

Specificities of Caries on Root Surface

Nailê Damé-Teixeira[a] · Clarissa Cavalcanti Fatturi Parolo[b] · Marisa Maltz[b]

[a]University of Brasilia, Brasilia, and [b]Federal University of Rio Grande do Sul, Porto Alegre, Brazil

Abstract

Variations in organic and inorganic composition and morphology may determine different susceptibilities of root surfaces to caries. Subsequent to gingival recession, root surfaces become exposed and those areas where Sharpey's fibers system was once inserted into the cementum are converted into canals for microbial penetration. In the presence of a cariogenic root biofilm, the fermentable carbohydrate from diet is converted into organic acid, and the root caries lesion is initiated in the exposed root site. We will revisit here the structural, biochemical, and histopathological specificities of root caries. Likewise enamel, the root surface exchange minerals with oral fluids, resulting in a subsuperficial root caries lesion. After mineral loss, the collagen is degraded and the lesion progresses. The specificities regarding the critical pH for demineralization of root hard tissues, the influence of cementum loss for lesion progression, and the organic matrix degradation will be discussed in this chapter. The tissue-related phenomena would create lesion with a unique histopathology. Active and arrested root carious lesions will be discussed through the gradual development from the cementum to dentin.

Introduction

Caries lesions located on the root surface have diagnostic and treatment specificities. Root caries is qualitative and substantially different from coronal caries. To effectively manage root carious lesions, the understanding of its basic characteristics is crucial. In addition to the topographic features, the composition and structure of root surfaces are singular. In this chapter, we will review the biochemical and histopathology of root caries, and the structural specificities of the root surface niche, which make the root caries a very specific event. The knowledge of root caries etiopathogenesis might provide meaningful information for the development of future preventive and efficient treatment strategies.

Dental Tissues and Peculiarities of Root Sites

Tissues that comprise dental and periodontal structures have singular characteristics when compared to other tissues in the organism. This singularity reflects in the specific mechanisms by which frequent mineral changes with oral fluids occur, the particular microbiota that colonize these structures, and the de-remineralization process. Physiological and functional characteristics provide the dental structures a complex identity. Two main parts constitute a tooth: the crown, which is responsible for the masticatory function, and the root, which provides teeth anchorage in the alveolar bone. The crown is classified into 2 portions, the anatomic crown, that is, the part of the tooth covered by enamel, and the clinical crown, the portion of a tooth that is above the gingival margin. The root surface is covered by cementum. If the cementum is not protected by the gingiva, it is easily abraded exposing the dentin to the external environment. Differences in topography, morphology, composition, and structure of root surfaces are observed when compared to the anatomic crown. Unlike the anatomic crown, which requires a well-mineralized strong covering tissue (enamel), a tissue that anchors periodontal fibers on the root surface (cementum) and the exposed dentin has other specificities.

Dental Hard Tissues and Their Composition

The composition of inorganic and organic contents differs per tissue and it reflects the properties of both. Enamel has a higher inorganic content (~90% prismatic crystals); it is durable and stronger than any other hard tissues in the body. On the contrary, cementum is constituted by 45–50% inorganic contents and 50% organic contents of its dry mass, basically collagen type I [1, 2]. Similar to cementum, dentin has a complex structural composition, containing more organic material than enamel. On the basis of wet weight, the composition of dentin is approximately 70% inorganic materials, 18% organic materials, and 12% water [3]. This organic content confers to root hard tissues more resilience than enamel.

Although the inorganic content of all hard tooth tissues consists of hexagonal crystals comprised of hydroxyapatite, $Ca_{10}[PO_4]_6[OH]_2$, the mineral content of the root surface is lower, and the crystal size is smaller than that in the enamel [2, 4]. In enamel, crystals are 100 nm long and 40 nm wide. Crystals are also highly oriented in enamel than in dentin. In dentin, crystals are 50 nm long and 20 nm wide. The mature crystals in cementum have similar size as in dentin and the crystallinity of the mineral component is lower in cementum than any other hard tissue [2].

The hydroxyapatite is not chemically pure but contains other minerals. Some ion substitution could occur in the inorganic content such as the hydroxyl substitution for fluoride, causing a considerable variation in apatite properties and a decrease in solubility. It has been shown that magnesium and carbonate contents of dentin/cementum are greater than those of enamel (~6.2 and ~1.2%, respectively) [2, 5], which could confer more solubility for crystals in both root hard tissues than in the anatomic crown covering tissue (enamel) due to the combination of phosphorus as $Mg_3[PO_4]_2$. This fact was corroborated by Hoppenbrouwers et al. [6] who developed demineralization in enamel and in both root hard tissues (dentin/cementum) by exposure to a buffer solution of pH 5.0. The authors showed that the root hard tissues are more soluble than the enamel.

Dental Hard Tissues and Their Morphology and Structure

Regarding the morphology and structure of tissues from anatomic crown and dental root, there are some peculiarities and variances to be discussed. The enamel is an avascular and acellular tissue, and it is permanently susceptible to several physicochemical changes when in contact with oral fluids. Due to its high mineral content, enamel has physical properties such as smoothness, transparency, friability, and translucency. On the contrary, the dental root tissues, dentin/enamel, apart from having a lower mineral content, exhibit a remarkable amount of organic components, such as collagen fibers

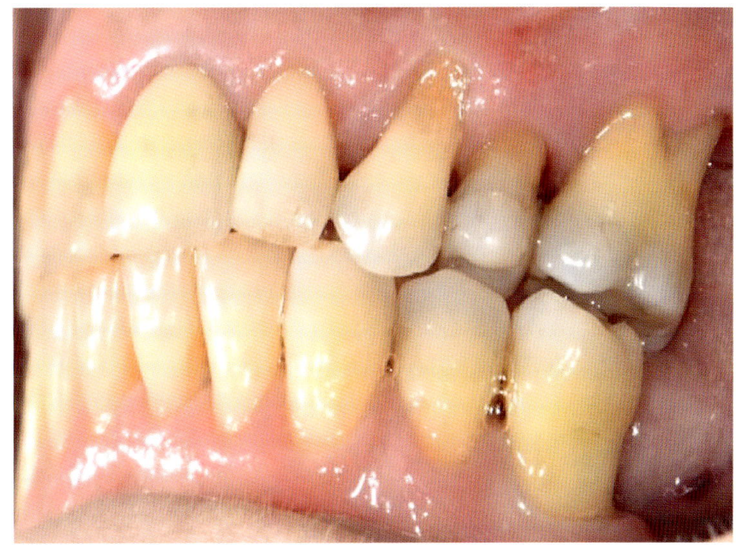

Fig. 1. Gingival recession associated with inadequate tooth brushing and periodontal disease, with cervical abrasion. Recession is associated with severe insertion loss.

and fibrils. In addition, the calcified matrix of dentin is permeated by tubules that host the cytoplasmic processes of odontoblasts. Thus, a very important characteristic of dentin is the capacity to continuously form dentin as secondary (when tooth becomes functional as a daily deposit) and tertiary dentin (as a reaction to an external aggression), but enamel does not have a regenerative capacity [1] (see Goldberg et al. [3] for more information).

Two types of cementum have been distinguished. The acellular type is characterized by a uniform mineralization and is found at the cervical, two-thirds of the root surface. The cellular cementum covers the apical third of the root surface and the furcation area in molars. The acellular cementum is composed of a very fibrous matrix of well-oriented collagen fiber bundles (Sharpey's fibers), promoting anchorage points for the periodontal ligament. The cementum thickness varies according to the region, and it increases in thickness towards the teeth apex [2]. Incremental lines are observed due to their layered formation [2]. Although cementum is considered as a part of teeth, it is not a dental structure, as its embryonary origin is the dental follicle, and not the enamel organ or dental papilla that is the embryonary origin of enamel, dentin, and pulp.

Gingival Recession and Exposition of Root Hard Tissues to Oral Environment

Gingival recession is the apical migration of the gingival margin by the gradual loss of periodontal insertion. As the gingival margin recedes the cementum-enamel junction, the cementum becomes exposed. The gingiva recedes by periodontal disease, as a result of inappropriate biofilm control procedures [7–10]. Gingival recession seems to occur with a characteristic intra-oral distribution pattern. Teeth with a prominent position in the jaw possess a high risk to lost attachment and to develop recession [9, 11]. Figure 1 shows a clinical case of gingival recession.

The cementum-enamel junction is highly irregular and represents a particular area, difficult to toothbrush, and a biofilm stagnation area [12]. This structure represents the cementum-to-enamel bonding line and can be present in 3 different forms: (1) edge-to-edge contact of cementum and enamel (most common in pre molars), (2) a small cementum line

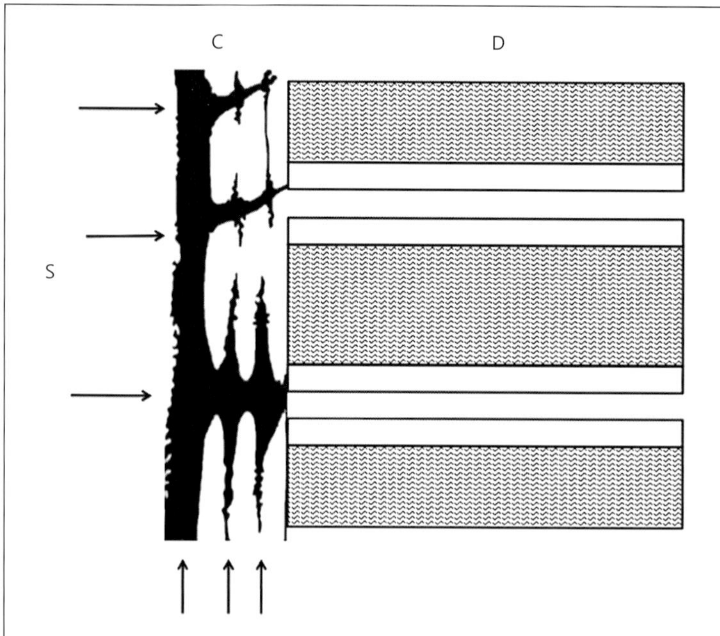

Fig. 2. Scheme of cementum canals for biofilm invasion: canals of Sharpey's fibers (horizontal arrows) and incremental lines (vertical arrows). C, cementum; D, dentin; S, surface. Adapted from Consolaro [14].

overlapping the enamel (most common in molars), (3) an exposed dentin area not covered by enamel or by cementum [13]. Once the root is exposed, a new ecological niche will be formed on the root surface. This surface, which used to be an anaerobic microenvironment underneath the gingival tissue, becomes an aerobic microenvironment with variable nutrient availability. The gingival crevicular fluid, a serum-like exudate, for example, is in contact with the root tissue and it can be exploited as a source of nutrient for microorganisms established in that niche. The microbiota composition also would change in the biofilm due to the microenvironment change. This will be discussed in the chapter by Do et al., this volume, pp. 26–34.

After root exposition, regions where Sharpey's fiber systems were implanted are gradually exposed and converted into canals through which the microbial penetration may occur to gain the proximity to the tissue (Fig. 2) [14]. Furthermore, improper tooth brushing or periodontal treatment of root surfaces often damages or completely removes the cementum, thus exposing the dentin. It has been shown that the cementum and the dentin tubules are obliterated by mineral changes from oral fluids due to the de-remineralization process at the interface tooth and saliva/crevicular fluid [15].

Biochemistry and Histopathology of Root Caries

In the presence of a cariogenic root biofilm, the fermentable carbohydrate from diet is converted into organic acids, and the root caries lesion is initiated in the exposed root site. Most of the root lesions originate along the exposed cementum-enamel junction or on the cervical third of the root, that are areas covered by acellular cementum, as previously stated [15]. Currently, the root caries is defined as a process of 2 stages [16]. The first stage is characterized by mineral dissolution and the second one by the degradation of the organic matrix of the root surface [16]. Figure 3 represents a model of root caries

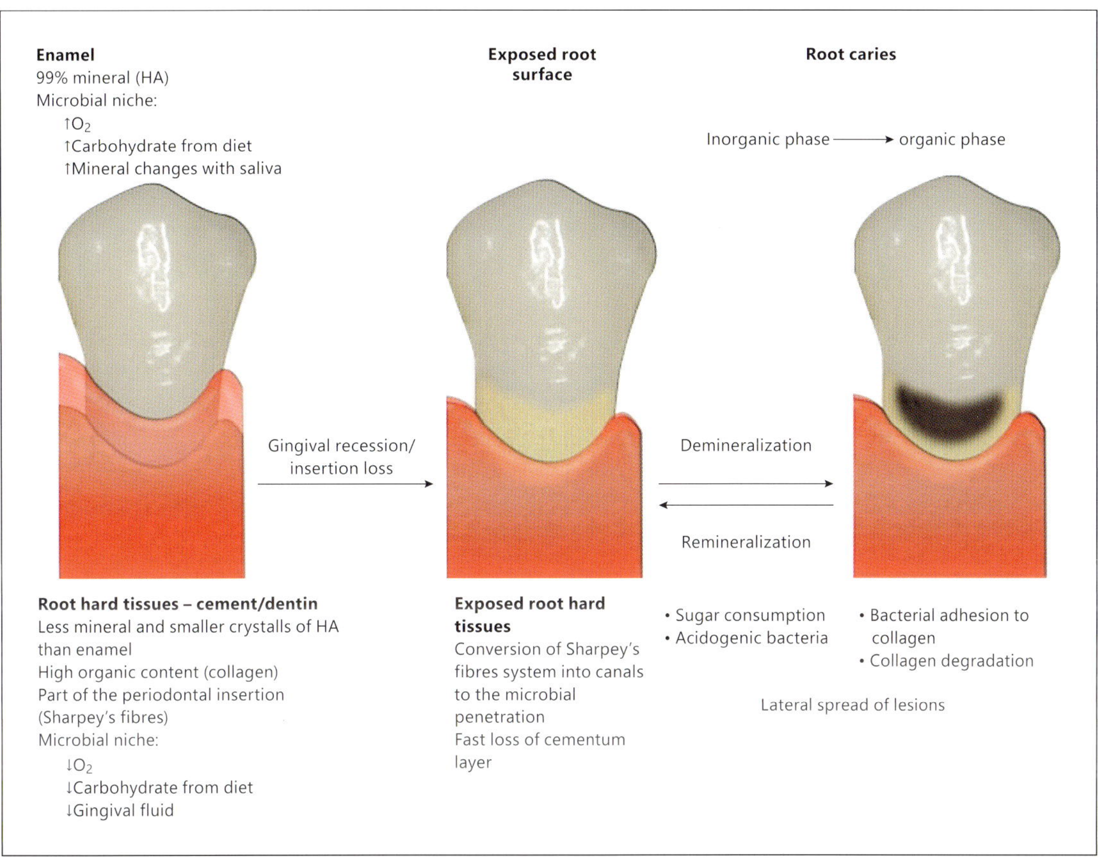

Fig. 3. A model of root caries specificities.

specificities. First, the microbial niche presents less oxygen and carbohydrate availability than the one above the enamel. Consequently, bacteria do not survive in an acidic environment. After gingival recession, this microenvironment changes and the microbiota may have to adapt to the new conditions above the cementum/dentin. In the presence of high amount of sugar, the mineral exchanges between oral fluids and tooth surface would lead to the demineralization of root hard tissues (inorganic phase of root caries). The progression of lesion would depend on the collagen degradation by endogenous or exogenous collagenases (organic phase of root caries) [16–18].

Mineral Dissolution
Biochemical differences of tooth hard tissues are reflected in the pattern of caries. The dissolution behaviors of cementum and dentin inorganic phases are similar. That is why most studies deal with them together, referring to chemical root mineral behavior as a whole. As discussed before, the root mineral appears to dissolve in buffer solutions saturated with respect to hydroxyapatite. For enamel, the critical pH is about 5.4. The critical pH for the root hard tissues has been estimated to range from about 6.8 to 6.0 [4]. More recently, Shellis [19] by studying the root lesion formation has confirmed that the solubility of the mineral of root

tissues is higher than that of hydroxyapatite, but indicated that such solubility is probably lower than suggested by Hoppenbrouwers et al. [4], ranging from 5.66 to 5.08. Critical pH represents the equilibrium between tooth mineral and dental plaque fluid. It means that the mineral of the root is more soluble than that of the enamel; therefore, it is much easier to demineralize the root surface in comparison to enamel. Some types of carbohydrates that are safe for enamel would be cariogenic for root surfaces, for example, sweeteners containing lactose as a bulking agent may be cariogenic to cementum/dentin [20–22]. Likewise, it has been proposed that the digestion of starch products by dental biofilm bacteria [23, 24] would be sufficient to cause root caries but not sufficient to cause enamel caries. Starch alone showed no demineralization in enamel [25], while complex carbohydrates such as starch contribute to the caries of the dentin/cementum [23]. Also, the association with starch and sucrose enhanced the sucrose effect in demineralization in both enamel [25] and dentin [26]. This fact could be associated with the digestion of starch by surface-adsorbed amylase [26].

Organic Matrix Degradation

The progression of caries lesions implicates in the degradation of the collagen matrix in the root hard tissues. The collagen protein family is characterized by the presence of proline-rich tripeptide "Gly-X-Y," forming a triple helix of polypeptide chains in which the glycine residue is positioned in the center [27]. The collagen type I, the most common in dentin, is a heterotrimer structure. The collagen structure contributes to the molecular stabilization and mechanical properties of the dentin. Only a specific group of proteases, the collagenases, would be able to degrade native collagen. The triple-helix is interrupted at its internal structure in the aqueous phase prior to the proteolytic degradation by the digestion of the amino group at a "Gly-Leu" bond. It may cause intramolecular flexibility and allow specific proteolytic cleavage [27].

Dental caries occurs in the mouth not by continuous demineralization but by alternating demineralization and remineralization. The exposed collagen is broken down, and the collagen content could be denatured during the second stage of caries process [16]. It was suggested that collagen matrix degradation could only be possible after demineralization and the reason is that the substrate is not approachable for collagenases in the mineralized tissue [16]. Furthermore, using a small-angle x-ray scattering for assessing the components of carious and sound extracted tooth, researchers showed that during the initial stages or only mild demineralization, a significant part of the collagen network is conserved in abundance and orientation [28]. It corroborates with the theory that collagen degradation is delayed with respect to the demineralization in root caries.

The demineralized collagen serves as a scaffold for colonizing bacteria [16]. Ultrastructural studies of root caries suggested that invading bacteria produce acids that demineralize the dentin [29–31]. Besides demineralization, bacteria could be also involved in matrix degradation. This is discussed in detail in the chapter by Do et al. (this volume, pp. 26–34).

The etiopathogenesis of root caries also involves some important response of the host tissues to the caries attack. Some endogenous collagenases have been shown to be involved in the dentin degradation [17, 18, 32]. Matrix metalloproteinases, a zinc-dependent endopeptidase group, are able to cleave the denatured collagen. They have a function in tissue development and repair and in pathological processes as well. Fibril-forming collagens I, II, and III are cleaved by some matrix metalloproteinases, that are secreted in their inactive forms; however, they are automatically activated under acidic conditions (around pH 4.5) [33]. The role of endogenous enzymes in root caries is addressed in the chapter by Boukpessi et al. (this volume, pp. 35–42).

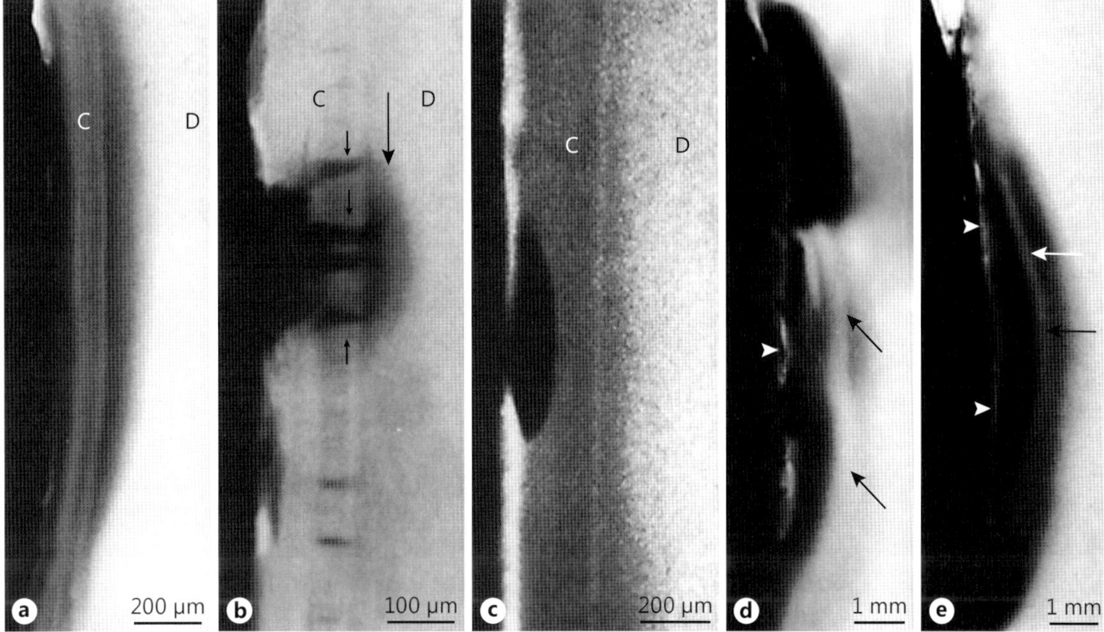

Fig. 4. Three patterns of demineralization of initial cementum lesions (**a–c**) and 2 patterns of advanced root caries lesions (**d**, **e**) proposed by Schüpback et al. [15, 34].

Histopathology of Root Caries

The mineral dissolution and the organic matrix degradation of the root surface will lead to lesion formation and progression. The treatment for root caries is achievable and lesions can be arrested. The arrest of an active lesion can be achieved by non-operative treatment (change in the environmental condition of the dental biofilm covering the lesion and fluoride treatment). The dentin/pulp organ responds to the cariogenic attack with an increased mineral deposition deep within the tissue. Furthermore, tertiary dentin can be formed corresponding to the involved tubules. The study of established root caries lesions in different stages of progression would explain how caries initiate and progress and, also, how it may become arrested. The histopathology of active and arrested root carious lesions was studied by Schüpbach et al. [15, 34, 35]. The gradual development of the caries lesions is shown from the cementum to the underlying dentin.

Lesions in Cementum

Clinically, the initial root caries lesion could be presented as a single lesion or multiple lesions. In microradiographs, 3 types of demineralization could be observed (Fig. 4a–c) [15]. Type "a" is the most prevalent one and corresponds to a uniform demineralization of cementum and underlying dentin. It is possible to observe accentuated lines in the cementum (it will be discussed later); type "b" was observed when microcavities were present in the root surface. Radially oriented radiolucent strips between the bottom of the cavity in the cementum and the cementum-dentin junction were observed. In dentin, a halo-like radiolucency at the end of the strips was present. Type "c" corresponds to a uniform demineralization of cementum and dentin with the maintenance of mineralized surface layer (10–30 μm) interrupted by a defined halo-like area of demineralization.

In this early stage of the carious process, a stepwise demineralization of the cementum occurs

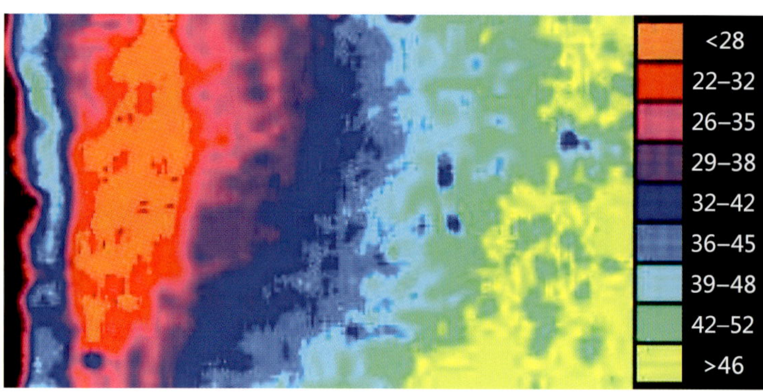

Fig. 5. Subsurface pattern of root caries lesions with mineral distribution of Ca + P. Wavelength dispersive spectrometry (WDS) was used to measure line intensities from Ca and P lines. Root caries lesions imaged by backscattered electron correlate to the Ca and P WDS profiles, that is, blue-green images correspond to higher amounts of Ca and P, while orange-red-purple zones represent lower amounts of these elements [37].

along fractures, which seemed to follow the incremental lines of cementum. Sometimes, small clefts traverse the cementum and extend into peripheral dentin. These clefts become bigger with the developing lesion and may serve as an entry point for bacterial penetration (Fig. 2). It is possible to observe enlarged clefts extending from the surface into the cementum filled with microorganisms. Other studies confirm that root surfaces become invaded by bacteria at an early stage of the caries process [15, 31].

Root hard tissues are highly reactive in the oral environment. Likewise in enamel, the root surface exchange minerals with oral fluids, resulting in a higher mineral content in the surface layer, as a result of demineralization-remineralization processes [16, 36]. In the early stages of root caries, minerals are dissolved following a gradient from the outer surface to dentin. A hypermineralized surface layer is a common feature in root caries similar to enamel caries. The mineral that is dissolved can precipitate underneath the cariogenic biofilm forming a thin protective layer (10–30 μm) [29]. Figure 5 [37] shows the gradient of calcium and phosphate from root caries lesion formed in situ. Under the mineralized surface layer, an area that corresponds to the body of the lesion presents a lower mineral composition. Figure 6 [37] shows a subsurface caries lesion on the root surface. A laminar pattern of the cementum, showing 2 well-mineralized surface layers (bands) is also observed. The remineralization can be observed in the surface layer of the lesion and along the lesion forming bands.

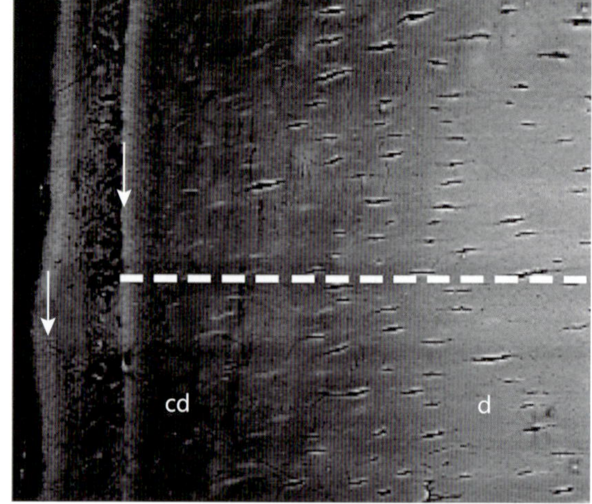

Fig. 6. Subsurface lesion on root surface with lamination. Backscattered electron image of the root, showing 2 well-mineralized surface layers (arrows), a demineralized zone in the carious dentin (cd) and sound dentin (d) [37].

The presence of cementum and its relation to caries progression or lesions depth has been discussed in the literature. It was proposed by McIntyre et al. [38] that the removal of the cementum layer accelerated the initial rate of root caries lesion progression. Most in vitro studies evaluate root caries formation with and without cementum [38, 39]. For Shellis [19], the process of gridding creates a smear layer and a subsurface region of mechanical damage, which are more vulnerable to dissolution [19]. However, there are no differences in the solubilities of cementum and dentin [16, 19, 34, 40]. From the clinical point of view, intact cement will be present in few situations once abrasion, tooth brushing or scaling removes it. The underlying dentin is sometimes the root tissue exposed to the oral cavity.

Root caries is different from coronal caries in terms of lesion shape. While in enamel caries lesion develops deep, in root surfaces it occurs laterally. It is common to observe a larger but thinner lesion. The possible explanation for this lateral spread is related to several factors: the presence of gingival crevicular fluid, thickness of bacterial deposits, and exposure to salivary flow [16] and the tooth tissue structure. Thinner biofilms may have easy access to salivary clearance of metabolites, reducing the acidity of the biofilm. Gingival crevicular fluid may also act as a modulatory agent in root caries because of its neutral to weakly alkaline pH. Besides, the accessibility to salivary flow allows a remineralization process and prevents the demineralization in depth [16]. While in the enamel demineralization follows the prism direction, the bacterial penetration in the cementum and dentin occurs along fractures, which seemed to follow the incremental lines of cementum contributing to the lateral lesion spreading.

Initial Lesion in Dentin

In the initial lesion in dentin, a step-wise destruction of dentin was observed. Areas of progressive dentin destruction could be distinguished from areas of further destruction. Halo-like areas extended into dentin. As in lesions where the cementum is kept, mineralized layers could also be found in dentin lesions. The initial penetration of microorganisms occurred following multiple clefts perpendicular to the surface. Eventually, clefts fused forming microcavities filled with microorganisms. In a subsequent process, bacteria could invade tubules [14, 15].

Advanced Lesions in Dentin

Two patterns of advanced lesions were observed (Fig. 4d, e) [35]. Pattern "d" (Fig. 4d) is characterized by multiple enlarged lesions that extend in depth along exposed root surfaces with halo-like areas covered by a radiolucent surface layer. Radiodense layers bordering the radiolucent area towards the inner dentin were also observed. Pattern "e" (Fig. 4e) presented only one radiolucent area extending the saucer-shape into the dentin. Mineralized layers at the surface and in the deep parts of the lesions were observed and it could be related to the intermittent process of caries and/or mineral re-precipitation [34, 41].

In advanced lesions, intertubular dentin is almost completely demineralized. The demineralization of the intertubular dentin occurs, forming microcavities that are further enlarged. Subsequently, bacteria are able to move deeper towards the open dentinal tubules, eventually infecting them. In advanced lesions, it is common to observe microorganisms inside dentin tubules and their side-branches. The invasion of dentin occurs initially along the dentinal tubules and then progress by a lateral spread into the partially demineralized intertubular dentin. Peritubular dentin is also affected by caries in advanced lesions. Nevertheless, signs of remineralization were also observed. In the surface layer, we can observe small needle-like crystals and in dentinal tubules mineral deposits occluding the lumen. Root carious lesion can be arrested despite dentin contamination once the external biofilm is controlled [31].

Arrested Lesions

Arrested lesions show pronounced surface abrasion. Interestingly, arrested root caries lesions were almost completely mineralized. Dentin tubules near the surface were packed with ghosts of microorganisms and granular crystals as well. In dentin, tubular sclerosis was observed. Granular crystals occluded tubular lumen, and intertubular dentin was also mineralized. This is a clear view of the reparative potential of the pulp/dentin organ in root caries [35].

Conclusion

- Tissues that form the root structures of the tooth have singular characteristics when compared to enamel. These characteristics may change the response of each of the dental tissues to cariogenic challenges;
- Critical pH has been estimated at 6.7 for root surface. However, recently it has been demonstrated to be lower and closer to the enamel critical pH (5.66–5.08). This understanding allows us to prevent and control root caries in an easier way;
- Lesion shape is different from coronal caries: while in enamel caries lesion develops in deep, in root surfaces it occurs laterally;
- Bacterial invasion occurs at an earlier stage in root caries compared to enamel caries. The tissue bacterial invasion does not prevent the control of active lesions once the external biofilm is controlled. Furthermore, dentin reaction as sclerosis and tertiary dentin control caries development;
- Root caries is developed in a 2-stage process. The first stage is characterized by mineral dissolution and the second one, by the degradation of the organic matrix of the root surface.

Acknowledgements

We gratefully thank Dr. Sergio Kiyoshi Ishikiriama (University of São Paulo, Bauru, Brazil), who kindly authorized the use of the tooth illustration in Figure 3.

References

1 Abou Neel EA, Aljabo A, Strange A, Ibrahim S, Coathup M, Young AM, et al: Demineralization-remineralization dynamics in teeth and bone. Int J Nanomedicine 2016;11:4743–4763.

2 Bosshardt DD, Selvig KA: Dental cementum: the dynamic tissue covering of the root. Periodontol 2000 1997;13:41–75.

3 Goldberg M, Kulkarni AB, Young M, Boskey A: Dentin: structure, composition and mineralization. Front Biosci (Elite Ed) 2011;3:711–735.

4 Hoppenbrouwers PM, Driessens FC, Borggreven JM: The mineral solubility of human tooth roots. Arch Oral Biol 1987;32:319–322.

5 Driessens FC: Mineral aspects of dentistry. Monogr Oral Sci 1982;10:1–215.

6 Hoppenbrouwers PM, Driessens FC, Borggreven JM: The vulnerability of unexposed human dental roots to demineralization. J Dent Res 1986;65:955–958.

7 Kassab MM, Cohen RE: The etiology and prevalence of gingival recession. J Am Dent Assoc 2003;134:220–225.

8 Merijohn GK: Management and prevention of gingival recession. Periodontol 2000 2016;71:228–242.

9 Sarfati A, Bourgeois D, Katsahian S, Mora F, Bouchard P: Risk assessment for buccal gingival recession defects in an adult population. J Periodontol 2010; 81:1419–1425.

10 Serino G, Wennström JL, Lindhe J, Eneroth L: The prevalence and distribution of gingival recession in subjects with a high standard of oral hygiene. J Clin Periodontol 1994;21:57–63.

11 Baelum V, Fejerskov O, Karring T: Oral hygiene, gingivitis and periodontal breakdown in adult Tanzanians. J Periodontal Res 1986;21:221–232.

12 Beighton D, Lynch E, Heath MR: A microbiological study of primary root-caries lesions with different treatment needs. J Dent Res 1993;72:623–629.

13 Schroeder HE, Scherle WF: Cemento-enamel junction – revisited. J Periodontal Res 1988;23:53–59.

14 Consolaro A: [Carie Dentaria: Histopatologia e Correlacoes Clinico-Radiograficas] [in Portuguese]. Sao Paulo, FOB, 1996.

15 Schüpbach P, Guggenheim B, Lutz F: Human root caries: histopathology of initial lesions in cementum and dentin. J Oral Pathol Med 1989;18:146–156.

16 Takahashi N, Nyvad B: Ecological hypothesis of dentin and root caries. Caries Res 2016;50:422–431.

17 Tjäderhane L, Larmas M: A high sucrose diet decreases the mechanical strength of bones in growing rats. J Nutr 1998; 128:1807–1810.

18 Tjäderhane L, Buzalaf MA, Carrilho M, Chaussain C: Matrix metalloproteinases and other matrix proteinases in relation to cariology: the era of 'dentin degradomics'. Caries Res 2015;49:193–208.

19 Shellis RP: Formation of caries-like lesions in vitro on the root surfaces of human teeth in solutions simulating plaque fluid. Caries Res 2010;44:380–389.

20 Aires CP, Tabchoury CP, Del Bel Cury AA, Cury JA: Effect of a lactose-containing sweetener on root dentine demineralization in situ. Caries Res 2002;36: 167–169.

21 Lingström P, Birkhed D: Effect of buccal administration of a lactose-containing nitroglycerin tablet (Suscard) on plaque pH. Scand J Dent Res 1994;102:324–328.

22 Giongo FC, Mua B, Parolo CC, Carlén A, Maltz M: Effects of lactose-containing stevioside sweeteners on dental biofilm acidogenicity. Braz Oral Res 2014;28:pii: S1806-83242014000100237.

23 Lingström P, van Houte J, Kashket S: Food starches and dental caries. Crit Rev Oral Biol Med 2000;11:366–380.

24 Neff D: Acid production from different carbohydrate sources in human plaque in situ. Caries Res 1967;1:78–87.

25 Ribeiro CC, Tabchoury CP, Del Bel Cury AA, Tenuta LM, Rosalen PL, Cury JA: Effect of starch on the cariogenic potential of sucrose. Br J Nutr 2005;94:44–50.

26 Botelho JN, Villegas-Salinas M, Troncoso-Gajardo P, Giacaman RA, Cury JA: Enamel and dentine demineralization by a combination of starch and sucrose in a biofilm – caries model. Braz Oral Res 2016;30:pii:S1806-83242016000100250.

27 Gelse K, Pöschl E, Aigner T: Collagens – structure, function, and biosynthesis. Adv Drug Deliv Rev 2003;55:1531–1546.

28 Deyhle H, Bunk O, Müller B: Nanostructure of healthy and caries-affected human teeth. Nanomedicine 2011;7:694–701.

29 Kawasaki K, Featherstone JD: Effects of collagenase on root demineralization. J Dent Res 1997;76:588–595.

30 Frank RM, Steuer P, Hemmerle J: Ultrastructural study on human root caries. Caries Res 1989;23:209–217.

31 Nyvad B, Fejerskov O: An ultrastructural study of bacterial invasion and tissue breakdown in human experimental root-surface caries. J Dent Res 1990;69: 1118–1125.

32 Toledano M, Nieto-Aguilar R, Osorio R, Campos A, Osorio E, Tay FR, et al: Differential expression of matrix metalloproteinase-2 in human coronal and radicular sound and carious dentine. J Dent 2010;38:635–640.

33 Ricard-Blum S: The collagen family. Cold Spring Harb Perspect Biol 2011; 3:a004978.

34 Schüpbach P, Guggenheim B, Lutz F: Histopathology of root surface caries. J Dent Res 1990;69:1195–1204.

35 Schüpbach P, Lutz F, Guggenheim B: Human root caries: histopathology of arrested lesions. Caries Res 1992;26: 153–164.

36 Nyvad B, Fejerskov O: Assessing the stage of caries lesion activity on the basis of clinical and microbiological examination. Community Dent Oral Epidemiol 1997;25:69–75.

37 Volkweis A, Maltz M: [Análise do Conteúdo Mineral de Lesões de Cárie Radicular Desenvolvidas in situ Através da Técnica de Microssonda Eletrônica] [thesis in Portuguese]. Porto Alegre, Federal University of Rio Grande do Sul, 2000.

38 McIntyre JM, Featherstone JD, Fu J: Studies of dental root surface caries. 2: the role of cementum in root surface caries. Aust Dent J 2000;45:97–102.

39 Dietz W, Kraft U, Hoyer I, Klingberg G: Influence of cementum on the demineralization and remineralization processes of root surface caries in vitro. Acta Odontol Scand 2002;60:241–247.

40 Dung TZ, Liu AH: Molecular pathogenesis of root dentin caries. Oral Dis 1999; 5:92–99.

41 Schüpbach P, Guggenheim B, Lutz F: Human root caries: histopathology of advanced lesions. Caries Res 1990;24: 145–158.

Nailê Damé-Teixeira
Department of Dentistry, Faculty of Health Science, University of Brasilia
Campus Universitário Darcy Ribeiro,
Asa Norte, Brasília, DF 70910-900 (Brazil)
E-Mail nailedame@hotmail.com

Carrilho MRO (ed): Root Caries: From Prevalence to Therapy.
Monogr Oral Sci. Basel, Karger, 2017, vol 26, pp 26–34 (DOI: 10.1159/000479304)

Root Surface Biofilms and Caries

Thuy Do[a] · Nailê Damé-Teixeira[b] · Monika Naginyte[a] · Philip D. Marsh[a]

[a]Division of Oral Biology, School of Dentistry, University of Leeds, Wellcome Trust Brenner Building, St James's University Hospital, Leeds, UK; [b]Department of Dentistry, Cariology, University of Brasilia, Brasilia, Brazil

Abstract

Following gingival recession, which increases with age, the root surface becomes exposed, creating new environments for microbial colonization and biofilm formation. The formation of root surface biofilms is influenced by the availability and composition of saliva and gingival crevicular fluid; they provide components for the conditioning film (acquired root surface pellicle) and also act as a source of nutrients. The early bacterial colonizers of the root surface are similar to those found on the enamel, and Gram-positive species such as *Streptococcus sanguinis*, *S. oralis*, *S. mitis*, and *Actinomyces* species predominate. The root surface has a lower mineral and higher organic content than enamel, and so is more vulnerable to demineralization. The characterization of the microbiota associated with root surface lesions is still ongoing. Traditional culture-based studies have implicated species such as mutans streptococci, lactobacilli, bifidobacteria, and *Actinomyces* species, while molecular-based studies have provided evidence for a more complex microbiota with many Gram-negative and anaerobic bacteria being detected in addition to the more conventional cariogenic organisms. Ecological concepts have been applied to explain the microbial etiology of root caries. The acidic environment generated from the fermentation of dietary sugars selects saccharolytic bacteria that can preferentially grow and metabolize under low pH conditions, and then proteolytic Gram-negative species are selected when the dentin is exposed and collagen and other proteins become accessible to be catabolized. These species act in concert to degrade the inorganic and organic components of the dental tissues.

Introduction

The germ theory of disease established by Koch and Pasteur in the late 19th century led to a revolution in new approaches to disease diagnosis, treatment, and prevention. However, investigations into the microbial etiology of root caries only began in the 1960s with experiments carried out on animals, which found that certain species of *Actinomyces* were capable of inducing the disease in pathogen-free rodents [1–3]. Early studies of the microbiota associated with root caries suggested that disease-implicated bacteria include Actinomyces, streptococci, enterococci, staphylococci, neisseria, lactobacilli species and *Rothia denticariosa*. These studies eventually led to the proposal of the specific plaque hypothesis which suggests that disease was caused by a few members of resident microbiota. However, it became clear following increased reports of the occurrence of disease in the apparent absence of these recognized pathogens that the concerted action of a polymicrobial community may be needed to drive dysbiosis, as proposed in the "non-specific plaque hypothesis." The "ecological plaque hypothesis," first proposed by Marsh [4], combines key concepts from the first 2 hypotheses, but emphasized the functional specificity of disease displayed by an enrichment of particular species, with relevant properties, in response to a change in environmental conditions.

A lower salivary flow rate, a common occurrence in the elderly, is one of the factors that promotes favorable conditions for a change in the microbiota, and predisposes sites to the development of caries. Once root surfaces are exposed, the cementum, which has a structure and biochemical composition distinct to that of the enamel, becomes vulnerable to physical abrasion and is susceptible to demineralization, often exposing the dentin. The cementum and dentin are less mineralized than enamel and are composed of higher proportions of organic materials such as collagen [5, 6], which has an impact on the microbiology of the caries process. The bacterial invasion of the cementum and dentin is accelerated by the metabolic activities of the biofilm, which break down the tissues [7]. The aim of this chapter is to explore the composition of the root surface biofilm in health and disease and to describe how lesion development is a process driven by the degradation of organic and inorganic host tissues by the biofilm community.

Influence of Saliva and Gingival Fluid on the Root Surface Biofilm

Saliva and gingival crevicular fluid (GCF) play a major role in determining the composition of dental biofilms that develop on the root surface. Both fluids contain a diverse array of proteins and glycoproteins that can (a) bind to cementum or exposed dentin, and act as a conditioning film that influences microbial colonization and biofilm formation, (b) act as primary sources of nutrients for the attached micro-organisms, and (c) influence the local pH by means of their buffering properties, while (d) the flow of both fluids will remove loosely attached microbes and deliver components of the host defenses, which restrict microbial growth.

As soon as dental surfaces are exposed to the oral environment, molecules in oral fluids are rapidly adsorbed to form a conditioning film (also termed the acquired pellicle). After being held reversibly near the root surface by electrochemical forces, adhesins on the surfaces of microorganisms interact with molecules in the conditioning film on cementum, and the outcome determines whether permanent attachment occurs. The major constituents of dental pellicles include glycoproteins, phosphoproteins, and lipids; specific examples include amylase, statherin, proline-rich peptides, mucins, and an array of antimicrobial proteins and host defense factors [8]. Enzymes from both the host and oral bacteria can be detected in dental pellicles; these enzymes remain active and can modify the structure of the pellicle [9]. Bacterially derived glucosyltransferases in the pellicle can synthesize glucans and directly influence bacterial colonization by acting as receptors for streptococci. The pellicle on exposed root surfaces contains more plasma proteins compared to enamel [10], and these may influence the pattern of biofilm formation. Although streptococci are the early colonizers of both enamel [11, 12] and root surfaces [12], *Actinomyces* species have been more frequently isolated from mature biofilms taken from exposed root surfaces at sites with periodontitis [10], and root surface biofilms also contain Gram-negative bacteria (see below).

The main sources of nutrients for the microorganisms attached to the root surface are the proteins and glycoproteins present in saliva and GCF. Host proteins are broken down by the concerted action of multiple microbial peptidases and proteases while glycoprotein catabolism requires the sequential removal of terminal sugars from oligosaccharide side chains that decorate and protect the protein backbone. Individual oral bacteria lack the full repertoire of glycosidases and proteases needed to fully break down these structurally complex molecules and, as a result, numerous metabolic collaborations and interdependencies develop between species with complementary enzyme profiles [13–15] (also reviewed by [16, 17]). Important consequences of these interdependencies are that individual species avoid direct competition for specific nutrients, and any pH changes following their metabolism are slow and small; both of these features promote the establishment of diverse microbial communities that are resilient to minor changes in environmental conditions, so that their composition remains relatively stable over time. The provision of an array of host proteins and glycoproteins by both oral fluids will also support the growth of more fastidious bacteria, including Gram-negative anaerobic or capnophilic proteolytic species such as *Prevotella*, *Fusobacterium*, *Capnocytophaga*, *Campylobacter*, and *Selenomonas* spp. [18–20]. Saliva and GCF also act as buffers, and would help maintain the pH around neutrality, which contributes to the establishment of stable and diverse microbial communities. Paradoxically, in addition to being a source of nutrients for dental bacteria, saliva and GCF also deliver components of the innate and adaptive host defenses, and these will also modulate the growth and activity of the developing root surface biofilms.

Development of Plaque Biofilms on Sound Root Surfaces

Root surfaces are initially covered by a conditioning film (the acquired root surface pellicle), composed of proteins and glycoproteins from saliva and GCF (see above). The stages of biofilm formation on enamel surfaces also apply to root surfaces; these involve the adhesion of microorganisms onto the acquired pellicle through a series of complex interactions, from weak electrostatic forces to specific molecular binding between bacterial adhesins and their corresponding receptors found on the pellicle, as mentioned before. Detailed reviews have described the succession of microbes colonizing the tooth [21, 22]. According to in situ studies, sound root and enamel surfaces are colonized by similar pioneer species [12], with non-mutans streptococci (e.g., *S. sanguinis*) and *Actinomyces* spp. constituting the majority of the bacterial species found in sound root surface biofilms [23–25].

Clinically, sound and carious root lesion surfaces are similar to supragingival plaque covering enamel in that the overall balance of de- and remineralization is controlled by the microbial activity in the plaque [21, 22]. A dynamic stability exists when the production of acids by some bacteria is negated by metabolic processes of other species within the plaque bringing the pH back towards neutrality, hence balancing the de- and remineralization processes. It has been found that this homeostasis is maintained by key organisms such as members of the non-mutans streptococci group (e.g., *S. sanguinis*, *S. oralis*, and *S. mitis*) and *Actinomyces* spp. [26, 27]. The metabolic activities of these bacteria result in an oscillating pH within the root surface biofilm. Each step along the caries development and progression line can be stopped, even during the cavitation stage, as long as the microbial metabolic processes are controlled.

Microbiology of Root Surface Caries

The increased consumption of refined sugars has undeniably had an impact on human oral and gut microbiome. In the mouth, acidification occurs as a result of the metabolism of dietary carbohydrates by the microbial populations within biofilms at various oral sites. The frequent intake of fermentable carbohydrates in the diet results in an increase in the abundance of certain species favored by low pH conditions, while others may be inhibited or eliminated. Persistence of such conditions causes an imbalance in both the composition of the biofilm and the de- and remineralization process, triggering the development of caries lesions. The basis of the ecological plaque hypothesis concept, proposed by Marsh [4, 28] and extended by Takahashi et al. [22, 27, 29], explains the microbial dynamics within dental plaque following sugar metabolism and its effect on the caries process. The concept emphasizes that changes to the local oral environment (e.g., regular exposure of plaque to conditions of low pH) can drive the selection of previously minor components of the dental biofilm that prefer such conditions. It has been proposed that the caries process could be divided into 3 distinct phases: (a) the "dynamic stability stage" where the metabolic activities of certain members of the plaque microbiota cause the pH to decrease, but homeostatic mechanisms help maintain a balance of the de- and remineralization process of the enamel and root surfaces; (b) the "acid adaptation stage" where the population of aciduric (acid-tolerating) non-mutans microbes increases due to a breakdown of homeostasis and contribute to lesion initiation; (c) the "aciduric stage" which occurs if these acidic conditions are not reversed; the non-mutans species may be progressively replaced by even stronger aciduric species such as the mutans streptococci, lactobacilli, and bifidobacteria whose metabolic activities further decrease the pH of the microenvironment. This situation facilitates the progression of the lesion. The microbiota composition decreases in diversity during these early stages of lesion development, shaped by the selective pressure, providing ideal conditions for aciduric and acidogenic strains to establish themselves as the dominant species in the biofilm.

The current understanding of the microbial etiology of root caries remains limited compared to other oral diseases [18, 19]. Early experiments on root caries used animals and found that certain species of *Actinomyces* and streptococci were able to cause root caries in gnotobiotic rodents [1, 30]. Subsequent human studies aimed to compare the microbiota of sound and carious root surface biofilms. According to early culture-dependent studies, mutans streptococci were found to form a third of the total microbiota of cavitated dentin lesions suggesting that these species play a major role in caries progression. However, in later stages of caries, other species such as lactobacilli, *Prevotella,* and *Bifidobacterium* species were found to be more prevalent [1, 31, 32].

The microbiota associated with root caries lesions has been found to be distinct from that of enamel caries [33], and further studies found it to be much more complex [24]. Indeed, microorganisms as diverse as *Bifidobacterium*, *Rothia*, *Veillonella*, enterococci, anaerobic Gram-negative rods, and *Candida albicans* have been detected [34]. There is evidence that the microorganisms associated with the development of root caries are not as dependent on refined carbohydrates as those from coronal caries [35]. This may be due to the differences in the structure and composition of these tissues, as well as the microenvironmental conditions, for example, dentinal lesions provide a wider range of nutrients, and drive an increase in the diversity of the associated microbial populations [36, 37].

Culture studies have also investigated the mechanism of sugar metabolism in both mutans and non-mutans streptococci, and determined that they can store excess sugars either intracellularly as polysaccharides or extracellularly as glucans. Mutans streptococci and lactobacilli are also able to tolerate and grow under the acidic conditions generated from sugar metabolism. This is an important survival strategy, giving them competitive advantages over other

Table 1. Bacterial species commonly detected in root caries, based on culture-independent approaches

Bacterial species	References
Actinomyces spp./*Actinomyces* clone IP073	[38]
Atopobium spp., *Olsenella* spp.	[38]
Bifidobacterium breve	[39]
Bifidobacterium subtile	[39]
Dialister invisus	[38, 40]
Enterococcus faecalis	[38, 40]
Lactobacillus spp./*L. casei*/*L. paracasei*/*L. rhamnosus*	[38, 41]
Olsenella profusa	[18]
Oribacterium spp.	[18]
Prevotella multisaccharivorax	[18, 38]
Propionibacterium acidifaciens	[18]
Propionibacterium spp. strain FMA5a	[38]
Pseudoramibacter alactolyticus	[40–42]
Selemonas spp. clone CS002 (Mitsuokella spp. HOT 131)	[38, 40]
Scardovia inopicata	[39]
Selemonas spp. strain GAA14 (Veillonellaceae oral taxon 155)	[38]
Streptococcus mutans	[18, 38, 42]

species. One of the features of some non-mutans streptococci is their possession of an arginine deiminase system allowing them to utilize arginine alone or arginine contained in proteins. This particular proteolytic pathway produces ammonia and carbon dioxide, releasing one ATP molecule, hence contributing to the neutralization of the environmental pH in plaque, and proving that these bacteria are able to use proteins found in saliva and GCF as an energy source [16]. Most mutans streptococci, which are acidogenic and aciduric in nature, have not been found to possess this pathway system, but they are instead equipped with various other pathways specializing in sugar metabolism. Mutans streptococci are, therefore, less competitive in the biofilms of clinically sound enamel and root surfaces, and hence have a lower abundance.

Numerous survival strategies have been established by the communities found on root surface. They are able to exploit the resources available, including unique glycolytic systems and physiological mechanisms allowing microorganisms to store metabolic compounds as energy reservoirs (e.g., use of polyphosphates, lactate) [22].

The emergence of molecular approaches to the investigation of dental plaque has led to several culture-independent studies on root caries to be carried out. Preza et al. [38] found that specific species including *Streptococcus mutans*, *Lactobacillus* spp., *Actinomyces*, *Atopobium*, *Olsenella*, *Pseudoramibacter*, *Propionibacterium*, and *Selemonas* could be considered etiological agents of root caries (Table 1). An extensive study of the supra-gingival microbiota in health and root caries carried out by Chen et al. [18] identified *Propionibacterium acidifaciens*, *Streptococcus mutans*, *Olsenella profusa*, *Prevotella multisaccharivorax*, and *Lactobacillus crispatus* as root caries pathogens. Other species such as *Delftia acidovorans*, *Bacteroidetes* (G-2) spp., *Lachnospiraceae* (G-3) spp., and *Prevotella intermedia* were found to be more prevalent in healthy samples, and therefore could be considered as health-associated species.

Role of Proteases in Caries Progression

The microbiota of root dentin biofilms is composed of a variety of aciduric and acidogenic organisms, as well as proteolytic bacteria such as *Prevotella* and *Propionibacterium* species [22, 41], all producing different organic acids rendering the lesions heterogeneous in terms of pH levels [40, 42]. This varying pH landscape is likely to be the result of the metabolism of a variety of saccharolytic species producing lactic acid, combined with the production of weaker acids from the utilization of lactic acid as an energy source by other organisms such as *Veillonella*. Proteolytic bacteria can also produce acids or ammonia from the catabolism of nitrogenous substrates, available either exogenously or from the dentin organic matrix [22, 39], and so can affect the biofilm pH in several ways.

Exposed root surfaces (cementum or dentin) are composed of almost 50% less mineral and higher proportions of organic materials than enamel, making them much more susceptible to physical damage and decay [43]. This difference in biochemical structure is reflected in the caries process. Indeed, microbial invasion of cementum and dentin tissues occurs at an early stage of the caries process, whereas in enamel caries, dentin is invaded only once and enamel is destroyed [22, 43]. The microbial activities within the root surface tissues are obviously dictated by the nutrients available (dietary sugars, proteins, and glycoproteins in saliva and GCF), leading to the accumulation of acidic by-products of metabolism. They will also be influenced by the presence of organic matrix (collagen) within the tissues. The ecological caries hypothesis for dentin and root caries was updated to take into account the roles of host and microbial proteases in the degradation of the dentin's organic matrix [22, 44, 45], and therefore their contribution to the development of cavities. Investigations into dentin structure and composition [46] have unveiled the presence of embedded host-derived proteases which can be activated under acidic conditions. Indeed, host-derived proteases such as matrix metalloproteinases (MMP-2, 3, 8, 9, and 20) and cysteine cathepsins (B and K) are present in the dentinal organic matrix [22, 47–53], and have been found to become activated once the cementum is degraded, and the dentin matrix exposed to the aqueous phase [22]. Microbial-derived proteases (collagenases, gelatinases, and peptidases) present in the saliva and GCF also contribute to the degradation of the dentinal matrix. The exposure of collagen molecules leads to an increase in their solubility through the action of host-derived collagenases and proteases, and solubilized collagen can be easily degraded at low pH levels [22].

As discussed in the chapter by Damé-Teixeira et al. (this volume, pp. 15–25), from a clinical point of view, the development of root caries may be considered a 2-stage process: the first stage is characterized by mineral dissolution and the second, by the degradation of the organic matrix of the root surface [22]. The demineralized collagen serves as a scaffold for colonizing bacteria and many studies have shown the presence of bacteria in early stages of caries [43, 54]. The degradation of the dentinal collagen matrix could be an important virulence trait (collagenase activity-dependent). Some studies found that EDTA-decalcified dentin is more resistant to bacterial collagenases [55] compared to acid-decalcified dentin [56, 57]. To understand the bacterial functions occurring within root caries lesions, a metatranscriptomic approach has been undertaken to investigate the gene expression of biofilms present in root caries lesions (Damé-Teixeira et al., unpublished data). Genes coding for collagenases showed high levels of expression in caries lesions: SMU_761 and SMU_759 (*Streptococcus mutans* UA159), VPAR_RS05935 and VPAR_RS05390 (*Veillonella parvula* DSM 2008), VEIDISOL_RS04770 (*Veillonella dispar* ATCC 17748), and LEBU_RS05040 (*Leptotrichia buccalis*; Fig. 1), thus confirming their important role in lesion development.

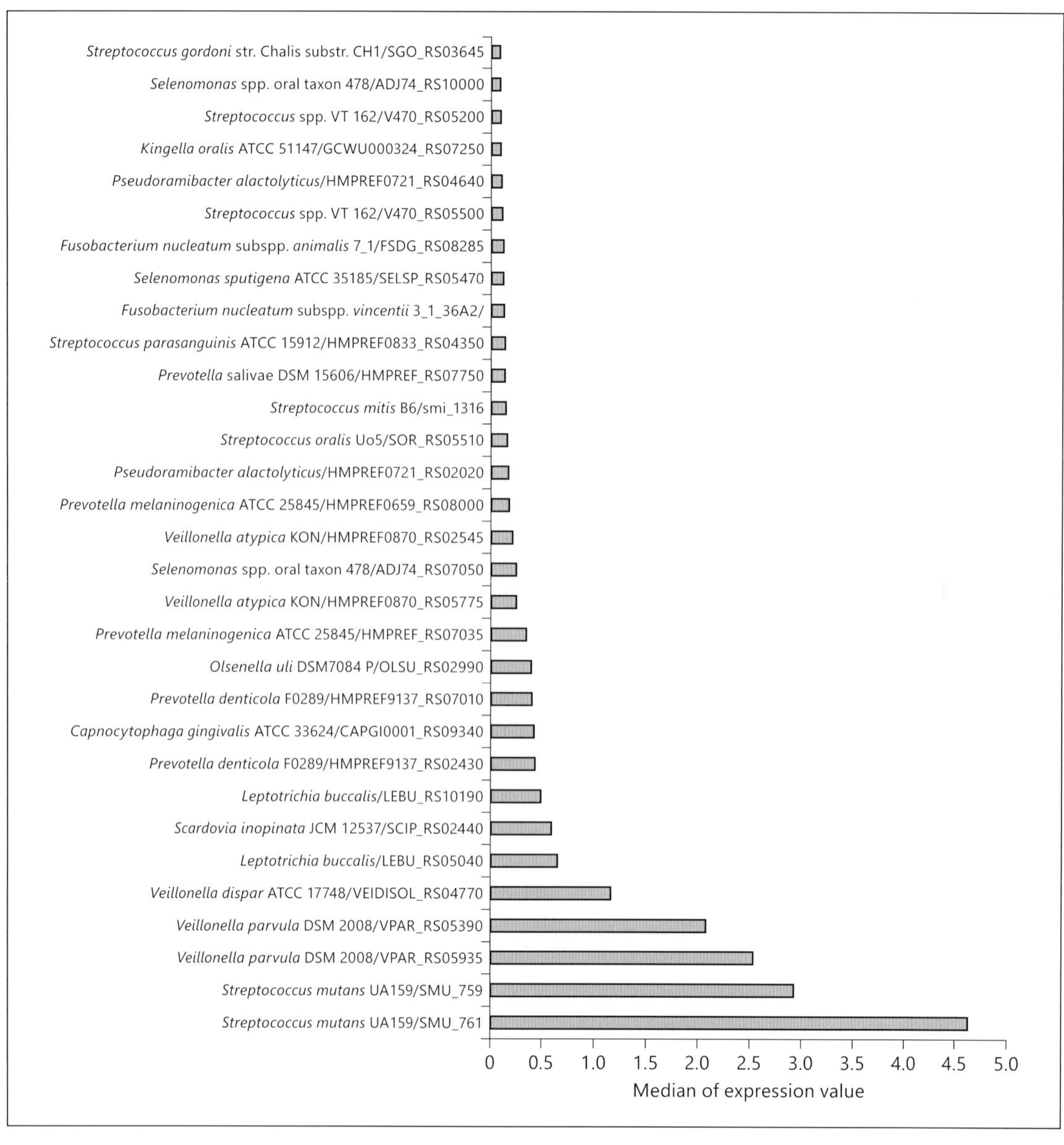

Fig. 1. The median of expression value (number of reads/number of mapped reads by sample*100,000) per gene coding for collagenases in root caries lesions (n = 9). Only the genes that had a median of expression value ">0.1" were displayed (Damé-Teixeira et al., unpublished data).

Conclusions

Epidemiological investigations of root caries have shown that the prevalence of root caries increases with age. Gingival recession exposes the root surface, which can be colonized by a range of mainly Gram-positive bacteria. However, a lack of good oral hygiene combined with high sugar intake and reduced salivary flow can induce a cascade of events where the biofilm builds up and matures, resulting in the acidification of the microenvironment and selection of acidogenic and aciduric bacteria. This leads to the breakdown of the natural de- and remineralization balance and favors net demineralization. Studies have demonstrated caries development and progression to be a complex process. The microbial species richness and complexity decrease during the initial caries process, perhaps reflecting the harshness of the acidic environment although some recent studies suggest that diversity may increase in dentinal caries when collagen and other host proteins are exposed and can act as substrates for proteolytic bacteria, many of which are Gram-negative and obligately anaerobic [37]. These species act in concert to degrade the inorganic and organic components of the dental tissues.

In conclusion, the following are key points concerning the role of microorganisms on root surface in health and disease:

- The pattern of biofilm formation on the root surfaces is influenced by the composition of the root surface pellicle, which contains more plasma proteins than the conditioning film on enamel.
- The early colonizers of a sound root surface are members of the non-mutans streptococci group and *Actinomyces* spp.
- Acidic conditions in the biofilm following sugar metabolism initially select for aciduric species, such as the mutans streptococci, lactobacilli, bifidobacteria, and *Actinomyces* spp.
- As the lesion develops into the dentin, the numbers of Gram-negative anaerobic and proteolytic bacteria increase as collagen and other host proteins and glycoproteins are exposed. The microbiota of the advanced lesion becomes more diverse, with saccharolytic and proteolytic activities which act in concert to degrade the inorganic and organic components of the dental tissues.

References

1 Jordan HV, Hammond BF: Filamentous bacteria isolated from human root surface caries. Arch Oral Biol 1972;17:1333–1342.

2 Jordan HV, Keyes PH: Aerobic, gram-positive, filamentous bacteria as etiologic agents of experimental periodontal disease in hamsters. Arch Oral Biol 1964;9:401–414.

3 Jordan HV, et al: Effect of lathyrogenic agents on dental caries in the rat. J Dent Res 1964;43:3–10.

4 Marsh PD: Microbial ecology of dental plaque and its significance in health and disease. Adv Dent Res 1994;8:263–271.

5 Bosshardt DD, Selvig KA: Dental cementum: the dynamic tissue covering of the root. Periodontol 2000 1997;13:41–75.

6 Goldberg M, et al: Dentin: structure, composition and mineralization. Front Biosci (Elite Ed) 2011;3:711–735.

7 Femiano F, et al: Dentin caries progression and the role of metalloproteinases: an update. Eur J Paediatr Dent 2016;17:243–247.

8 Lee YH, et al: Proteomic evaluation of acquired enamel pellicle during in vivo formation. PLoS One 2013;8:e67919.

9 Hannig C, Hannig M, Attin T: Enzymes in the acquired enamel pellicle. Eur J Oral Sci 2005;113:2–13.

10 Rüdiger SG, Dahlén G, Carlén A: Protein and bacteria binding to exposed root surfaces and the adjacent enamel surfaces in vivo. Swed Dent J 2015;39:11–22.

11 Heller D, Helmerhorst EJ, Oppenheim FG: Saliva and serum protein exchange at the tooth enamel surface. J Dent Res 2017;96:437–443.

12 Nyvad B, Kilian M: Microbiology of the early colonization of human enamel and root surfaces in vivo. Scand J Dent Res 1987;95:369–380.

13 Bradshaw DJ, Marsh PD: Effect of sugar alcohols on the composition and metabolism of a mixed culture of oral bacteria grown in a chemostat. Caries Res 1994;28:251–256.

14 ter Steeg PF, Van der Hoeven JS: Development of periodontal microflora on human serum. Microb Ecol Health Dis 1989;2:1–10.

15 ter Steeg PF, et al: Enrichment of subgingival microflora on human serum leading to accumulation of Bacteroides species, Peptostreptococci and Fusobacteria. Antonie Van Leeuwenhoek 1987;53:261–272.

16 Marsh PD, et al: Influence of saliva on the oral microbiota. Periodontol 2000 2016;70:80–92.

17 Marsh PD, Zaura E: Dental biofilm: ecological interactions in health and disease. J Clin Periodontol 2017;44(suppl 18):S12–S22.

18 Chen L, et al: Extensive description and comparison of human supra-gingival microbiome in root caries and health. PLoS One 2015;10:e0117064.

19 Preza D, et al: Diversity and site-specificity of the oral microflora in the elderly. Eur J Clin Microbiol Infect Dis 2009;28:1033–1040.

20 Schüpbach P, Osterwalder V, Guggenheim B: Human root caries: microbiota in plaque covering sound, carious and arrested carious root surfaces. Caries Res 1995;29:382–395.
21 Nyvad B: Microbial colonization of human tooth surfaces. APMIS Suppl 1993; 32:1–45.
22 Takahashi N, Nyvad B: Ecological hypothesis of dentin and root caries. Caries Res 2016;50:422–431.
23 Emilson CG, Klock B, Sanford CB: Microbial flora associated with presence of root surface caries in periodontally treated patients. Scand J Dent Res 1988; 96:40–49.
24 Van Houte J, et al: Association of the microbial flora of dental plaque and saliva with human root-surface caries. J Dent Res 1990;69:1463–1468.
25 van Houte J, Lopman J, Kent R: The predominant cultivable flora of sound and carious human root surfaces. J Dent Res 1994;73:1727–1734.
26 Marsh PD, Lewis MAO, Rogers H, Williams DW, Wilson M: Dental plaque; in Marsh and Martin's Oral Microbiology, Sixth Edition. Edinburgh, Elsevier, 2016.
27 Takahashi N, Nyvad B: Caries ecology revisited: microbial dynamics and the caries process. Caries Res 2008;42:409–418.
28 Marsh PD: Are dental diseases examples of ecological catastrophes? Microbiology 2003;149:279–294.
29 Takahashi N, Nyvad B: The role of bacteria in the caries process: ecological perspectives. J Dent Res 2011;90:294–303.
30 Sumney DL, Jordan HV: Characterization of bacteria isolated from human root surface carious lesions. J Dent Res 1974;53:343–351.
31 Bowden GH, et al: Association of selected bacteria with the lesions of root surface caries. Oral Microbiol Immunol 1990;5:346–351.
32 Shen S, et al: Bacterial and yeast flora of root surface caries in elderly, ethnic Chinese. Oral Dis 2002;8:207–217.
33 Syed SA, et al: Predominant cultivable flora isolated from human root surface caries plaque. Infect Immun 1975;11: 727–731.
34 Shen S, Samaranayake LP, Yip HK: Coaggregation profiles of the microflora from root surface caries lesions. Arch Oral Biol 2005;50:23–32.
35 Ellen RP, Banting DW, Fillery ED: Streptococcus mutans and Lactobacillus detection in the assessment of dental root surface caries risk. J Dent Res 1985;64: 1245–1249.
36 Rôças IN, et al: Microbiome of deep dentinal caries lesions in teeth with symptomatic irreversible pulpitis. PLoS One 2016;11:e0154653.
37 Simón-Soro A, Guillen-Navarro M, Mira A: Metatranscriptomics reveals overall active bacterial composition in caries lesions. J Oral Microbiol 2014;6:25443.
38 Preza D, et al: Bacterial profiles of root caries in elderly patients. J Clin Microbiol 2008;46:2015–2021.
39 Takahashi N: Oral microbiome metabolism: from "who are they?" to "what are they doing?". J Dent Res 2015;94:1628–1637.
40 Hojo S, et al: Acid profiles and pH of carious dentin in active and arrested lesions. J Dent Res 1994;73:1853–1857.
41 Aas JA, et al: Bacteria of dental caries in primary and permanent teeth in children and young adults. J Clin Microbiol 2008;46:1407–1417.
42 Hojo S, Takahashi N, Yamada T: Acid profile in carious dentin. J Dent Res 1991;70:182–186.
43 Schüpbach P, Guggenheim B, Lutz F: Human root caries: histopathology of advanced lesions. Caries Res 1990;24: 145–158.
44 Dayan D, Binderman I, Mechanic GL: A preliminary study of activation of collagenase in carious human dentine matrix. Arch Oral Biol 1983;28:185–187.
45 Tjäderhane L, et al: The activation and function of host matrix metalloproteinases in dentin matrix breakdown in caries lesions. J Dent Res 1998;77:1622–1629.
46 Tezvergil-Mutluay A, et al: Effect of phosphoric acid on the degradation of human dentin matrix. J Dent Res 2013; 92:87–91.
47 Boushell LW, et al: Distribution and relative activity of matrix metalloproteinase-2 in human coronal dentin. Int J Oral Sci 2011;3:192–199.
48 Buzalaf MA, Charone S, Tjäderhane L: Role of host-derived proteinases in dentine caries and erosion. Caries Res 2015; 49(suppl 1):30–37.
49 Mazzoni A, et al: Immunohistochemical identification of MMP-2 and MMP-9 in human dentin: correlative FEI-SEM/TEM analysis. J Biomed Mater Res A 2009;88:697–703.
50 Shimada Y, et al: Localization of matrix metalloproteinases (MMPs-2, 8, 9 and 20) in normal and carious dentine. Aust Dent J 2009;54:347–354.
51 Sulkala M, et al: The localization of matrix metalloproteinase-20 (MMP-20, enamelysin) in mature human teeth. J Dent Res 2002;81:603–607.
52 Tjäderhane L, et al: Matrix metalloproteinases and other matrix proteinases in relation to cariology: the era of 'dentin degradomics'. Caries Res 2015;49:193–208.
53 Toledano M, et al: Differential expression of matrix metalloproteinase-2 in human coronal and radicular sound and carious dentine. J Dent 2010;38:635–640.
54 Nyvad B, Fejerskov O: An ultrastructural study of bacterial invasion and tissue breakdown in human experimental root-surface caries. J Dent Res 1990;69: 1118–1125.
55 Konetzka W, Burnett G, Pelczar M: Bacterial hydrolysis of decalcified dentine. Brit D J 1956;100:156.
56 Armstrong WG: Further studies on the action of collagenase on sound and carious human dentin. J Dent Res 1958;37: 1001–1015.
57 Klont B, ten Cate JM: Susceptibility of the collagenous matrix from bovine incisor roots to proteolysis after in vitro lesion formation. Caries Res 1991;25: 46–50.

Thuy Do
Division of Oral Biology, School of Dentistry, University of Leeds
Wellcome Trust Brenner Building, St James' University Hospital, Beckett Street
Leeds LS9 7TF (UK)
E-Mail n.t.do@leeds.ac.uk

Carrilho MRO (ed): Root Caries: From Prevalence to Therapy.
Monogr Oral Sci. Basel, Karger, 2017, vol 26, pp 35–42 (DOI: 10.1159/000479305)

Endogenous Enzymes in Root Caries

Tchilalo Boukpessi[a, b] • Suzanne Menashi[a] • Catherine Chaussain[a, b]

[a]Dental School, University Paris Descartes Sorbonne Paris Cité, Laboratory EA2496 Orofacial Pathologies, Imaging and Biotherapies, Montrouge, and [b]AP-HP, Departments of Odontology, University Hospitals Bretonneau (PNVS) and Charles Foix (PSCF), Paris, France

Abstract

Similar to coronal caries, root caries results from a disequilibrium of the de-remineralization balance in favor of the demineralization process. It mainly involves a bacterial shift in favor of an increase in the proportion of acidogenic and aciduric bacteria. This process permanently damages the dental mineralized tissues, namely the dental cementum and dentin. In addition to the demineralization and exposure of the dentin or the cementum organic matrix, acid production by cariogenic bacteria induces the activation of endogenous (host-derived) enzymes within the dentin and saliva. These enzymes include matrix metalloproteinases and cathepsins. Once activated, these potent proteolytic enzymes collectively have the capacity to degrade all the components of the exposed organic dentin and cementum matrices. In this chapter, the description of the healthy cement and dentin organic matrices and their endogenous proteases will be followed by the role of these proteases in the root caries process.

Introduction

Both dentin and saliva contain endogenous (host-derived) proteases that collectively have the capacity to degrade all the components of the exposed organic dentin and cementum matrices during the carious process. In this chapter, healthy cementum and dentin organic matrices will be described with a special focus on their endogenous proteases. In a second part, the role of these proteases in the root caries process will be discussed.

Dental Cementum

The dental cementum, which covers the root surface, has been much less studied than bone and dentin but is generally compared to the bone [1]. Hence, the composition of cellular cementum and bone extracellular matrix (ECM) has been previously described and presents similar profiles of collagens, proteoglycans, phosphoproteins, and other components [1–5]. It mainly consists of a collagen type I scaffold associated with non-collagenous proteins (NCPs) including bone sialoprotein, dentin matrix protein 1, fibronectin, osteocalcin, osteonectin, osteopontin, tenascin, proteoglycans, proteolipids. It also contains several growth factors including the cementum growth factor that appears to be an insulin-like growth factor-like molecule [5]. The presence of endogenous proteases in the dental cementum has not yet been reported but we can hypothesize that, in view of the similarity with bone where these enzymes are highly expressed [6], they may also be expressed in the dental cementum.

Endogenous Enzymes in the Root Dentin

The root dentin ECM, similar to coronal dentin, mainly consists of a collagen type I scaffold (90%) [7, 8]. NCPs constitute the remaining 10% of the ECM and are a heterogeneous group of proteoglycans, phosphoproteins, glycoproteins, serum proteins, enzymes, and growth factors [9]. Similar to bone or cementum, some NCPs, either phosphorylated or non-phosphorylated, are associated with specific sites of collagen fibrils to regulate the mineralization process, controlling the nucleation and growth of hydroxyapatite crystals [10, 11]. A high concentration of dentin sialoprotein, which is encoded by the *DSSP* gene, distinguishes dentin from bone or dental cementum ECM [12].

Dentin contains matrix metalloproteinases (MMPs), which play an important role in matrix remodeling during dentinogenesis [13]. In humans, the 28 members of the MMP family are frequently divided into 6 groups – collagenases, gelatinases, stromelysins, matrilysins, membrane-type MMPs, and other MMPs – based on substrate specificity and homology. MMPs are secreted as inactive proenzymes (zymogens), in which the prodomain prevents the functional activity of the catalytic domain. Activation occurs when the prodomain bridge with the catalytic zinc (the "cysteine switch") is disrupted by prodomain cleavage by other MMPs, cysteine cathepsins or other proteinases, or chemically, such as pH changes [8, 13]. Once activated, MMPs display the optimum functional activity in a neutral environment, which is important in the carious context. The main MMPs identified in pulp, odontoblasts, and predentin/dentin compartments are the collagenase MMP-8, the gelatinases MMP-2 and MMP-9, stromelysin-1 (MMP-3), the MMP-2 activator MMP-14 (MT1-MMP), and MMP-13 [14–22]. TIMPs, their endogenous inhibitors were also detected in dentin ECM [15, 23]. MMP-2, which is the predominant MMP in sound dentin, is thought to play a key role during dentinogenesis [24], especially for basement membrane degradation [25–27]. At more advanced stages of dentinogenesis, MMP-2 and MMP-9 were found near the dentino-enamel junction [15, 28], and a strong gelatinase activity was detected by in situ zymography along the mantle dentin [29]. MMP-2 was isolated from mature human mineralized dentin matrix [30], and zymographically identified in demineralized dentin [31, 32], suggesting a potential role in dentin ECM degradation during the carious process [33, 34]. Studies have described a differential profile of localization and activity of the gelatinases in the different layers of human sound dentin [35, 36]. High levels of MMP-2 were observed in odontoblasts, where it co-localized with TIMP-2. It was also observed in the deep dentin and at the dentino-enamel junction [15]. MMP-9, which co-localized with TIMP-1, was also shown to decrease from the deep to the superficial dentin layer [35]. This gelatinase gradient, which may be important for dentinogenesis, may influence the rate of collagen degradation under pathological conditions, depending on the depth of the affected dentin.

Stromelysin-1 (MMP-3), which can degrade several substrates in the ECM, has been identified in predentin, where it was proposed to participate in the mineralization process by degrading CS/DS proteoglycans [37] and in dentin where it was shown localized within the intertubular dentin, along the collagen fibrils [17]. MMP-3 was identified in demineralized mature dentin in its active form, which may imply that it has the potential to degrade and disorganize the dentin matrix [14]. Indeed, when active, MMP-3 is able to cleave from the collagen scaffold several ECM components such as small proteoglycans (decorin, biglycan), as well as 4 members of the SIBLING family: dentin sialoprotein, matrix extracellular phosphoglycoprotein, bone sialoprotein, and osteopontin [14]. The release of proteoglycans by MMP-3, such as decorin, could result in a subsequent release of the sequestered cytokines which in turn may activate other MMPs, thus potentiating the degradation of the demineralized matrix [38, 39]. Hence, MMP-3 and also in concert with other MMPs may participate in peritubular and tertiary dentin formation, and in the release of dentinal growth factors which in turn would regulate defensive reactions in the pulp [8, 40–46].

More recently, another important family of proteases, the cysteine cathepsins, was identified in dentin [47, 48]. There are 11 human cysteine cathepsins, cathepsins B, C, F, H, K, L, O, S, V, X, and W. The majority of cathepsins are ubiquitously expressed in human tissues, but cathepsins K, W, and S show more restricted cell- or tissue-specific distribution [8]. Cysteine cathepsins participate intracellularly in diverse processes, such as normal protein turnover, pro-protein processing, and apoptosis. Extracellularly, they can contribute directly to the degradation of the ECM, and participate in proteolytic cascades that amplify the degradative capacity. Unlike MMPs, cysteine cathepsins have optimal activity in a slightly acidic pH, which may depend on the substrate [46, 49].

In addition to the dentin organic matrix, the dentinal fluid, which is derived from the pulp and fills the dentin tubules, also represents a source of MMPs and cysteine cathepsins in dentin. Indeed, MMP-2 has been identified in the dentinal fluid [50] and the dentin tubules were shown to display high gelatinolytic activity even in healthy teeth [51]. This suggests that these enzymes can participate and accelerate the destruction of dentin ECM.

Endogenous Enzymes in the Saliva

An additional contribution to the degradation of the root demineralized organic matrices (cementum and dentin) could result from the proteases contained in the saliva [32–34]. Saliva has been reported to contain several MMPs derived from both gingival crevicular fluid and salivary glands, and MMP-8 and MMP-9 are the most abundant salivary MMPs [32]. Salivary MMPs can efficiently degrade exposed dentin (or cementum) collagen matrix [34], which is the case for root caries where saliva has a direct access to the lesion [52]. Saliva also contains cysteine cathepsins [48], mainly cathepsin B [32]. In both saliva and dentinal fluid, the quantity and more importantly the activity of these enzymes appear to be greatly enhanced throughout the carious process [33, 41, 53].

Root Caries

Dental caries is a reversible disease of the calcified tissues of the tooth, characterized by demineralization and subsequent destruction of the organic substance of the tooth, eventually leading to cavitation. The progression of caries into the dentin requires bacterial invasion along the dentin-enamel junction or dentin-cementum junction. The surface of roots becomes exposed due to aging and more so by tooth wear and periodontal diseases. Mechanical instrumentation during scaling and root planning can also contribute to the disappearance of the cementum. Root dentin is also vulnerable to acidic dissolution because of its high critical pH for demineralization (6.2–6.4) [52]. Developing root surface caries is often manifested as lesion covering the broad surface of the entire root [54]. The acidic environment is created by cariogenic bacteria, exposing the dentin matrix. However, cariogenic bacteria cannot entirely degrade the dentin organic matrix after demineralization [2, 55]. In fact, bacterial collagenases can degrade the dentin matrix in a remineralization solution but not in a demineralization solution, suggesting that proteolysis related to bacteria may only occur during the remineralization phase. The optimum pH for bacterial enzyme activity is close to neutral, and this activity is directly reduced by the acidic pH [56]. Furthermore, studies have shown that bacteria collected from dentinal lesions created in situ were unable to degrade collagen in vitro [57]. Moreover, purified bacterial collagenases have low degrading activity in a very acidic environment [58, 59]. It can, therefore, be assumed that the cariogenic demineralization process initiated by the bacteria re-exposes endogenous MMPs and also potentially induces their activation through the acidity they create [34, 60], hence enabling further dentin matrix degradation. Low pH was suggested to cause a conformational change within the propeptide domain of the MMP that facilitates the cysteine switch, a critical step in the activation process [34]. Although the activated MMPs are stable in acidic pH, they can only be functional in neutral pH. Neutralization of acids can be achieved by the dentinal buffering mechanisms [61, 62] through the salivary buffer systems, thus allowing the pH-activated MMPs to cleave matrix components [34]. In addition, the phosphorylated proteins released from the collagen scaffold by bacterial acids could interact with TIMP-inhibited MMPs within the carious lesion and re-activate them, enhancing the degradation process [63].

Host Proteases and Root Caries

Host-derived MMPs that have the potential to be proteolytically active during the carious process include collagenases (MMP-1, MMP-8), gelatinases (MMP-2, MMP-9), and stromelysin (MMP-3) [14, 18, 33, 34, 64]. Along this line, dentin protein extracts obtained from the different dentin layers of decayed teeth were shown to have their gelatinase activity gradually increased from sound to the more infected dentin extracts (superficial soft carious lesion, inner soft carious lesion, affected dentin, sound dentin) [41]. These observations confirm that endogenous MMP-2 contained within the sound dentin is activated during the carious process. It has also been suggested by immunohistochemical observations that the endogenous MMP-2 level may be increased through the induction of MMP-2 synthesis in the presence of caries [53]. This was supported by a study showing that *MMP-2* and *TIMP-2* gene expressions were significantly upregulated in odontoblasts adjacent to the carious lesion [41].

Cysteine cathepsins may also participate in dentinal caries development. A previous study reported a stronger immunostaining of cathepsins B in carious dentin, observed in dentin tubules and in odontoblasts, when compared with sound dentin [48]. Cathepsin activity increases with increasing depth of the lesion, indicating the role of pulp tissue-derived enzymes [48]. This phenomenon may be caused by the influx of odontoblast- or pulp-derived enzymes via dentinal tubules. Hence, cysteine cathepsins B and K may participate in the carious process at least partly by activating latent MMPs. Cysteine cathepsins B and K seem to be involved in accelerating active caries lesions.

Based on current knowledge, it is not possible to determine with certainty the exact role and importance of salivary, dentin or pulp-derived (via dentinal fluid) enzymes in dentinal caries lesions. Saliva contains several MMPs, which have been experimentally shown to efficiently degrade exposed dentin collagen matrix [32, 34, 48]. Indeed, the incubation of demineralized dentin slabs with acid-pretreated saliva resulted in the degradation of the organic matrix [32]. As saliva bathes the root carious lesions, it is not surprising that the active form of MMP-9 was systematically detected by zymography performed on dentin extracts from several carious teeth [34]. Together these studies indicate that salivary MMPs may have a strong contribution to dentin matrix degradation during the caries process. Interestingly, it was also shown in this study that MMP activity in the saliva was higher in patients with active compared to chronic carious lesions [48]. Furthermore, high level of MMP-8 and MMP-9 in the outer carious layer compared to the inner (caries-affected) layer indicated that saliva was a source of these enzymes [65, 66].

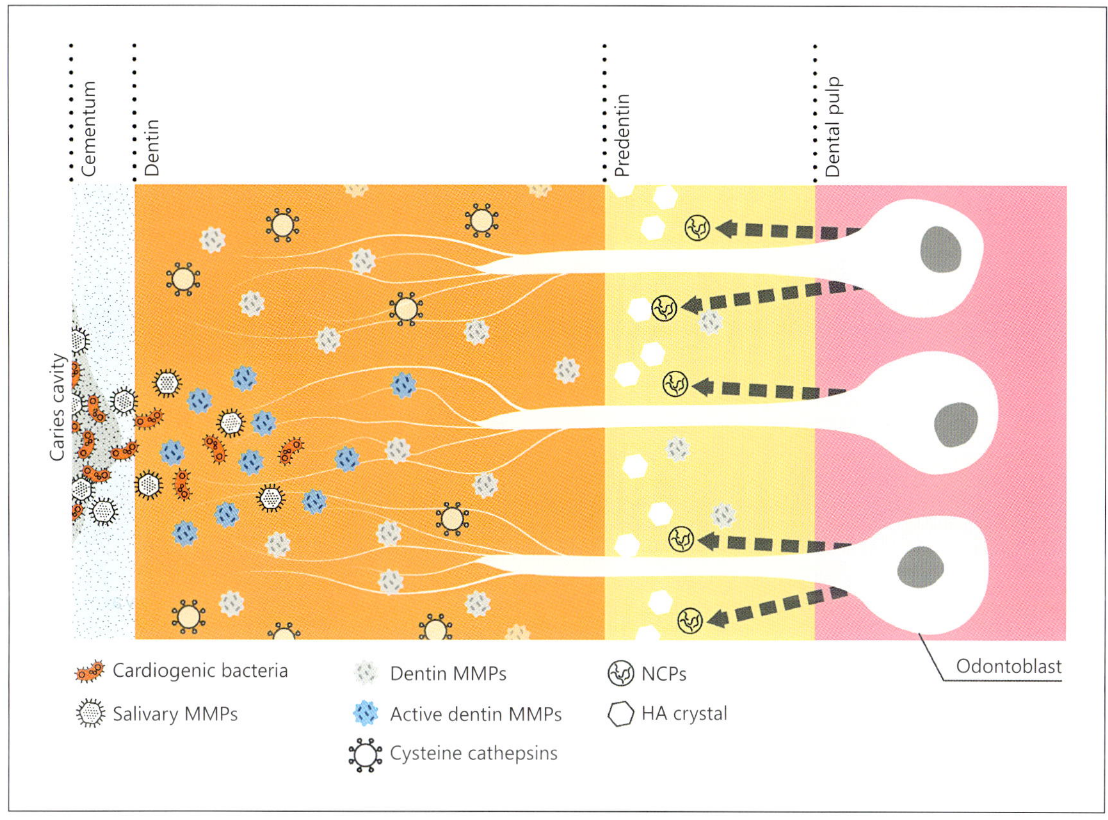

Fig. 1. Recapitulative schema of the role of host proteases in the root carious process.

Dentin Collagen Matrix during Caries

Dentin collagen matrix in caries-affected dentin has usually been considered to remain mostly intact, retaining its ability to remineralize even when up to half of the mineral content has been lost. However, Suppa et al. [39] demonstrated significantly reduced intact type I collagen and proteoglycans in caries-affected compared to normal dentin. Deyhle et al. [67] have suggested a significant correlation between the loss of mineral component and the loss of collagen periodicity. In fact, the statistically significant loss of minerals in caries-affected dentin is accompanied by a respective loss of collagen periodicity signal [67]. Since the collagen periodicity relates to the presence of terminal telopeptides next to the gap junction, the loss of telopeptides (seen as the loss of periodicity) may mean that intrafibrillar remineralization cannot occur, even though the total mineral loss is still relatively low [46]. As MMP-2 and MMP-9 and cysteine cathepsin K have telopeptidase activities, that is, they are able to cleave off the C-terminal end of the collagen molecule, dentin MMPs and cysteine cathepsins are considered responsible for the release of telopeptide fragments called ICTP (carboxy terminal telopeptides of type I collagen released by MMPs) and CTX (carboxy terminal telopeptides released by cathepsins). ICTP and CTX release has been used to highlight the degradation of demineralized dentin in many in vitro studies [68, 69]. Thus, these data suggest that dentin collagen may be prone to structural changes after mild demineralization in natural caries lesions.

Conclusions

Demineralized cementum and dentin organic matrices are exposed to degradation by endogenous (host-derived) proteases, mainly including MMPs and cysteine cathepsins (Fig. 1). Once activated, these potent enzymes have the capacity to degrade all the components of the ECM, dramatically enhancing the degradation process initiated by cariogenic bacteria. In contrast to coronal caries where dentin is protected by enamel, root caries progresses more rapidly due to the salivary MMPs, which have a direct access to the dental mineralized tissues. This easily initiates the degradation process once the cementum or dentin surface is demineralized by bacterial acids.

References

1 Zhao N, Foster BL, Bonewald LF: The cementocyte – an osteocyte relative? J Dent Res 2016;95:734–741.

2 Femiano F, Femiano R, Femiano L, Jamilian A, Rullo R, Perillo L: Dentin caries progression and the role of metalloproteinases: an update. Eur J Paediatr Dent 2016;17:243–247.

3 Cavuoti S, Matarese G, Isola G, Abdolreza J, Femiano F, Perillo L: Combined orthodontic-surgical management of a transmigrated mandibular canine. Angle Orthod 2016;86:681–691.

4 Nanci A, Bosshardt DD: Structure of periodontal tissues in health and disease. Periodontol 2000 2006;40:11–28.

5 Salmon CR, Giorgetti AP, Paes Leme AF, Domingues RR, Sallum EA, Alves MC, Kolli TN, Foster BL, Nociti FH Jr: Global proteome profiling of dental cementum under experimentally-induced apposition. J Proteomics 2016;141:12–23.

6 Pasternak B, Aspenberg P: Metalloproteinases and their inhibitors-diagnostic and therapeutic opportunities in orthopedics. Acta Orthop 2009;80:693–703.

7 Goldberg M, Smith AJ: Cells and extracellular matrices of dentin and pulp: a biological basis for repair and tissue engineering. Crit Rev Oral Biol Med 2004;15:13–27.

8 Tjäderhane L, Buzalaf MA, Carrilho M, Chaussain C: Matrix metalloproteinases and other matrix proteinases in relation to cariology: the era of 'dentin degradomics'. Caries Res 2015;49:193–208.

9 Goldberg M, Smith AJ: Cells and extracellular matrices of dentin and pulp: a biological basis for repair and tissue engineering. Crit Rev Oral Biol Med 2004;15:13–27.

10 Qin C, Baba O, Butler WT: Post-translational modifications of sibling proteins and their roles in osteogenesis and dentinogenesis. Crit Rev Oral Biol Med 2004;15:126–136.

11 Opsahl Vital S, Gaucher C, Bardet C, Rowe PS, George A, Linglart A, Chaussain C: Tooth dentin defects reflect genetic disorders affecting bone mineralization. Bone 2012;50:989–997.

12 D'Souza RN, Cavender A, Sunavala G, Alvarez J, Ohshima T, Kulkarni AB, MacDougall M: Gene expression patterns of murine dentin matrix protein 1 (Dmp1) and dentin sialophosphoprotein (DSPP) suggest distinct developmental functions in vivo. J Bone Miner Res 1997;12:2040–2049.

13 Visse R, Nagase H: Matrix metalloproteinases and tissue inhibitors of metalloproteinases: structure, function, and biochemistry. Circ Res 2003;92:827–839.

14 Boukpessi T, Menashi S, Camoin L, Tencate JM, Goldberg M, Chaussain-Miller C: The effect of stromelysin-1 (MMP-3) on non-collagenous extracellular matrix proteins of demineralized dentin and the adhesive properties of restorative resins. Biomaterials 2008;29:4367–4373.

15 Goldberg M, Septier D, Bourd K, Hall R, George A, Goldberg H, Menashi S: Immunohistochemical localization of MMP-2, MMP-9, TIMP-1, and TIMP-2 in the forming rat incisor. Connect Tissue Res 2003;44:143–153.

16 Mazzoni A, Pashley DH, Tay FR, Gobbi P, Orsini G, Ruggeri A Jr, Carrilho M, Tjäderhane L, Di Lenarda R, Breschi L: Immunohistochemical identification of MMP-2 and MMP-9 in human dentin: correlative FEI-SEM/TEM analysis. J Biomed Mater Res A 2009;88:697–703.

17 Mazzoni A, Papa V, Nato F, Carrilho M, Tjäderhane L, Ruggeri A Jr, Gobbi P, Mazzotti G, Tay FR, Pashley DH, Breschi L: Immunohistochemical and biochemical assay of MMP-3 in human dentine. J Dent 2011;39:231–237.

18 Sulkala M, Tervahartiala T, Sorsa T, Larmas M, Salo T, Tjäderhane L: Matrix metalloproteinase-8 (MMP-8) is the major collagenase in human dentin. Arch Oral Biol 2007;52:121–127.

19 Sulkala M, Pääkkönen V, Larmas M, Salo T, Tjäderhane L: Matrix metalloproteinase-13 (MMP-13, collagenase-3) is highly expressed in human tooth pulp. Connect Tissue Res 2004;45:231–237.

20 Sulkala M, Larmas M, Sorsa T, Salo T, Tjäderhane L: The localization of matrix metalloproteinase-20 (MMP-20, enamelysin) in mature human teeth. J Dent Res 2002;81:603–607.

21 Palosaari H, Ding Y, Larmas M, Sorsa T, Bartlett JD, Salo T, Tjäderhane L: Regulation and interactions of MT1-MMP and MMP-20 in human odontoblasts and pulp tissue in vitro. J Dent Res 2002;81:354–359.

22 Vidal CM, Tjäderhane L, Scaffa PM, Tersariol IL, Pashley D, Nader HB, Nascimento FD, Carrilho MR: Abundance of MMPs and cysteine cathepsins in caries-affected dentin. J Dent Res 2014;93:269–274.

23 Palosaari H, Pennington CJ, Larmas M, Edwards DR, Tjäderhane L, Salo T: Expression profile of matrix metalloproteinases (MMPs) and tissue inhibitors of MMPs in mature human odontoblasts and pulp tissue. Eur J Oral Sci 2003;111:117–127.

24 Bourd-Boittin K, Fridman R, Fanchon S, Septier D, Goldberg M, Menashi S: Matrix metalloproteinase inhibition impairs the processing, formation and mineralization of dental tissues during mouse molar development. Exp Cell Res 2005;304:493–505.

25 Sahlberg C, Reponen P, Tryggvason K, Thesleff I: Association between the expression of murine 72 kDa type IV collagenase by odontoblasts and basement membrane degradation during mouse tooth development. Arch Oral Biol 1992; 37:1021–1030.

26 Sahlberg C, Reponen P, Tryggvason K, Thesleff I: Timp-1, -2 and -3 show coexpression with gelatinases A and B during mouse tooth morphogenesis. Eur J Oral Sci 1999;107:121–130.

27 Heikinheimo K, Salo T: Expression of basement membrane type IV collagen and type IV collagenases (MMP-2 and MMP-9) in human fetal teeth. J Dent Res 1995;74:1226–1234.

28 Goldberg M, Septier D, Bourd K, Hall R, Jeanny JC, Jonet L, Colin S, Tager F, Chaussain-Miller C, Garabédian M, George A, Goldberg H, Menashi S: The dentino-enamel junction revisited. Connect Tissue Res 2002;43:482–489.

29 Pessoa JI, Guimarães GN, Viola NV, da Silva WJ, de Souza AP, Tjäderhane L, Line SR, Marques MR: In situ study of the gelatinase activity in demineralized dentin from rat molar teeth. Acta Histochem 2013;115:245–251.

30 Martín-de las Heras S, Valenzuela A, Overall CM: Gelatinase A in human dentin as a new biochemical marker for age estimation. J Forensic Sci 2000;45:807–811.

31 Mazzoni A, Mannello F, Tay FR, Tonti GA, Papa S, Mazzotti G, Di Lenarda R, Pashley DH, Breschi L: Zymographic analysis and characterization of MMP-2 and -9 forms in human sound dentin. J Dent Res 2007;86:436–440.

32 van Strijp AJ, Jansen DC, DeGroot J, ten Cate JM, Everts V: Host-derived proteinases and degradation of dentine collagen in situ. Caries Res 2003;37:58–65.

33 Chaussain-Miller C, Fioretti F, Goldberg M, Menashi S: The role of matrix metalloproteinases (MMPs) in human caries. J Dent Res 2006;85:22–32.

34 Tjäderhane L, Larjava H, Sorsa T, Uitto VJ, Larmas M, Salo T: The activation and function of host matrix metalloproteinases in dentin matrix breakdown in caries lesions. J Dent Res 1998;77:1622–1629.

35 Niu LN, Zhang L, Jiao K, Li F, Ding YX, Wang DY, Wang MQ, Tay FR, Chen JH: Localization of MMP-2, MMP-9, TIMP-1, and TIMP-2 in human coronal dentine. J Dent 2011;39:536–542.

36 Boushell LW, Kaku M, Mochida Y, Yamauchi M: Distribution and relative activity of matrix metalloproteinase-2 in human coronal dentin. Int J Oral Sci 2011;3:192–199.

37 Hall R, Septier D, Embery G, Goldberg M: Stromelysin-1 (MMP-3) in forming enamel and predentine in rat incisor-coordinated distribution with proteoglycans suggests a functional role. Histochem J 1999;31:761–770.

38 Imai K, Hiramatsu A, Fukushima D, Pierschbacher MD, Okada Y: Degradation of decorin by matrix metalloproteinases: identification of the cleavage sites, kinetic analyses and transforming growth factor-beta1 release. Biochem J 1997;322:809–814.

39 Suppa P, Ruggeri A Jr, Tay FR, Prati C, Biasotto M, Falconi M, Pashley DH, Breschi L: Reduced antigenicity of type I collagen and proteoglycans in sclerotic dentin. J Dent Res 2006;85:133–137.

40 Chaussain C, Boukpessi T, Khaddam M, Tjaderhane L, George A, Menashi S: Dentin matrix degradation by host matrix metalloproteinases: inhibition and clinical perspectives toward regeneration. Front Physiol 2013;4:308.

41 Charadram N, Farahani RM, Harty D, Rathsam C, Swain MV, Hunter N: Regulation of reactionary dentin formation by odontoblasts in response to polymicrobial invasion of dentin matrix. Bone 2012;50:265–275.

42 Mazzoni A, Tjäderhane L, Checchi V, Di Lenarda R, Salo T, Tay FR, Pashley DH, Breschi L: Role of dentin MMPs in caries progression and bond stability. J Dent Res 2015;94:241–251.

43 Muromachi K, Kamio N, Narita T, Annen-Kamio M, Sugiya H, Matsushima K: MMP-3 provokes CTGF/CCN2 production independently of protease activity and dependently on dynamin-related endocytosis, which contributes to human dental pulp cell migration. J Cell Biochem 2012;113:1348–1358.

44 Hannas AR, Pereira JC, Granjeiro JM, Tjäderhane L: The role of matrix metalloproteinases in the oral environment. Acta Odontol Scand 2007;65:1–13.

45 Tjäderhane L: The mechanism of pulpal wound healing. Aust Endod J 2002;28: 68–74.

46 Tjäderhane L, Nascimento FD, Breschi L, Mazzoni A, Tersariol IL, Geraldeli S, Tezvergil-Mutluay A, Carrilho MR, Carvalho RM, Tay FR, Pashley DH: Optimizing dentin bond durability: control of collagen degradation by matrix metalloproteinases and cysteine cathepsins. Dent Mater 2013;29:116–135.

47 Tersariol IL, Geraldeli S, Minciotti CL, Nascimento FD, Pääkkönen V, Martins MT, Carrilho MR, Pashley DH, Tay FR, Salo T, Tjäderhane L: Cysteine cathepsins in human dentin-pulp complex. J Endod 2010;36:475–481.

48 Nascimento FD, Minciotti CL, Geraldeli S, Carrilho MR, Pashley DH, Tay FR, Nader HB, Salo T, Tjäderhane L, Tersariol IL: Cysteine cathepsins in human carious dentin. J Dent Res 2011;90:506–511.

49 Turk V, Stoka V, Vasiljeva O, Renko M, Sun T, Turk B, Turk D: Cysteine cathepsins: from structure, function and regulation to new frontiers. Biochim Biophys Acta 2012;1824:68–88.

50 Zehnder M, Wegehaupt FJ, Attin T: A first study on the usefulness of matrix metalloproteinase 9 from dentinal fluid to indicate pulp inflammation. J Endod 2011;37:17–20.

51 Mazzoni A, Nascimento FD, Carrilho M, Tersariol I, Papa V, Tjäderhane L, Di Lenarda R, Tay FR, Pashley DH, Breschi L: MMP activity in the hybrid layer detected with in situ zymography. J Dent Res 2012;91:467–472.

52 Takahashi N, Nyvad B: Ecological hypothesis of dentin and root caries. Caries Res 2016;50:422–431.

53 Toledano M, Nieto-Aguilar R, Osorio R, Campos A, Osorio E, Tay FR, Alaminos M: Differential expression of matrix metalloproteinase-2 in human coronal and radicular sound and carious dentine. J Dent 2010;38:635–640.

54 Amer RS, Kolker JL: Restoration of root surface caries in vulnerable elderly patients: a review of the literature. Spec Care Dentist 2013;33:141–149.

55 Katz S, Park KK, Palenik CJ: In-vitro root surface caries studies. J Oral Med 1987;42:40–48.

56 Buzalaf MA, Hannas AR, Magalhães AC, Rios D, Honório HM, Delbem AC: pH-cycling models for in vitro evaluation of the efficacy of fluoridated dentifrices for caries control: strengths and limitations. J Appl Oral Sci 2010;18:316–334.

57 van Strijp AJ, van Steenbergen TJ, ten Cate JM: Bacterial colonization of mineralized and completely demineralized dentine in situ. Caries Res 1997;31:349–355.

58 Clarkson BH, Krell D, Wefel JS, Crall J, Feagin FF: In vitro caries-like lesion production by Streptococcus mutans and Actinomyces viscosus using sucrose and starch. J Dent Res 1987;66:795–798.

59 Kawasaki K, Featherstone JD: Effects of collagenase on root demineralization. J Dent Res 1997;76:588–595.

60 Sulkala M, Wahlgren J, Larmas M, Sorsa T, Teronen O, Salo T, Tjäderhane L: The effects of MMP inhibitors on human salivary MMP activity and caries progression in rats. J Dent Res 2001;80: 1545–1549.

61 Haapasalo M, Qian W, Portenier I, Waltimo T: Effects of dentin on the antimicrobial properties of endodontic medicaments. J Endod 2007;33:917–925.

62 Camps J, Pashley DH: Buffering action of human dentin in vitro. J Adhes Dent 2000;2:39–50.

63 Fedarko NS, Jain A, Karadag A, Fisher LW: Three small integrin binding ligand N-linked glycoproteins (SIBLINGs) bind and activate specific matrix metalloproteinases. FASEB J 2004;18:734–736.

64 Mazzoni A, Mannello F, Tay FR, Tonti GA, Papa S, Mazzotti G, Di Lenarda R, Pashley DH, Breschi L: Zymographic analysis and characterization of MMP-2 and -9 forms in human sound dentin. J Dent Res 2007;86:436–440.

65 Shimada Y, Ichinose S, Sadr A, Burrow MF, Tagami J: Localization of matrix metalloproteinases (MMPs-2, 8, 9 and 20) in normal and carious dentine. Aust Dent J 2009;54:347–354.

66 Hedenbjörk-Lager A, Bjørndal L, Gustafsson A, Sorsa T, Tjäderhane L, Åkerman S, Ericson D: Caries correlates strongly to salivary levels of matrix metalloproteinase-8. Caries Res 2015;49: 1–8.

67 Deyhle H, Bunk O, Müller B: Nanostructure of healthy and caries-affected human teeth. Nanomedicine 2011;7:694–701.

68 Tezvergil-Mutluay A, Mutluay M, Seseogullari-Dirihan R, Agee KA, Key WO, Scheffel DL, Breschi L, Mazzoni A, Tjäderhane L, Nishitani Y, Tay FR, Pashley DH: Effect of phosphoric acid on the degradation of human dentin matrix. J Dent Res 2013;92:87–91.

69 Osorio R, Yamauti M, Osorio E, Ruiz-Requena ME, Pashley D, Tay F, Toledano M: Effect of dentin etching and chlorhexidine application on metalloproteinase-mediated collagen degradation. Eur J Oral Sci 2011;119:79–85.

Catherine Chaussain
EA 2496, Orofacial Pathologies, Imaging and Biotherapies, Dental School
University Paris Descartes Sorbonne Paris Cité
1 rue Maurice Arnoux
FR–92120 Montrouge (France)
E-Mail catherine.chaussain@parisdescartes.fr

Carrilho MRO (ed): Root Caries: From Prevalence to Therapy.
Monogr Oral Sci. Basel, Karger, 2017, vol 26, pp 43–54 (DOI: 10.1159/000479306)

Root Surface Caries – Rationale Behind Good Diagnostic Practice

Ole Fejerskov[a] · Bente Nyvad[b]

Departments of [a]Biomedicine and [b]Dentistry and Oral Health, Faculty of Health, Aarhus University, Aarhus, Denmark

Abstract

Root surfaces, which with increasing age become exposed to dental biofilms, will react to the intermittent pH fluctuations at the interface between the biofilm and the cementum/dentin surface. If dental biofilm is left undisturbed in stagnation sites in the dentition, the underlying mineral surfaces may gradually develop dental caries characterized by a subsurface loss of mineral. In root surfaces, the demineralization is accompanied by microbial invasion of the cementum and dentin resulting in a pulpo-dentinal defense reaction. Most lesions progress slowly and experimental in situ studies as well as clinical studies document that the daily removal of the biofilm using fluoride toothpaste can arrest lesion progression. By applying this caries control measure, caries lesions can thus be transformed from active lesions to inactive lesions. The diagnostic characteristics of these types of lesions are mandatory to apply in daily clinical practice to avoid unnecessary restorative and antimicrobial treatments.

Introduction

With increasing age, gingiva recedes gradually and root surfaces become exposed to the oral environment in most individuals. Loss of attachment is associated with age but should not be seen as a consequence of aging. The presence of gingival recession in subjects with a good oral hygiene suggests that the etiology is multifactorial and involves anatomical and iatrogenic factors as well as factors associated with gingivitis and periodontitis (for a review, see [1]).

Root surfaces may be more vulnerable to mechanical damage than enamel surfaces because of differences in the structure and composition between the tissues. In populations with a tradition for regular oral hygiene procedures, the shallow layer of root cementum on the coronal part of the root is easily abraded away, exposing the dentin. This phenomenon is

1

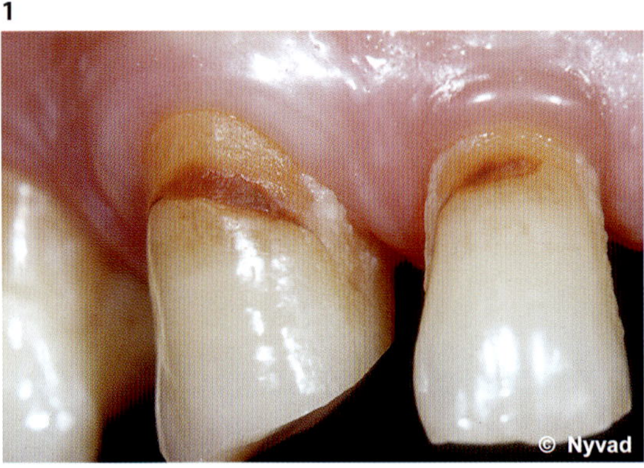

2

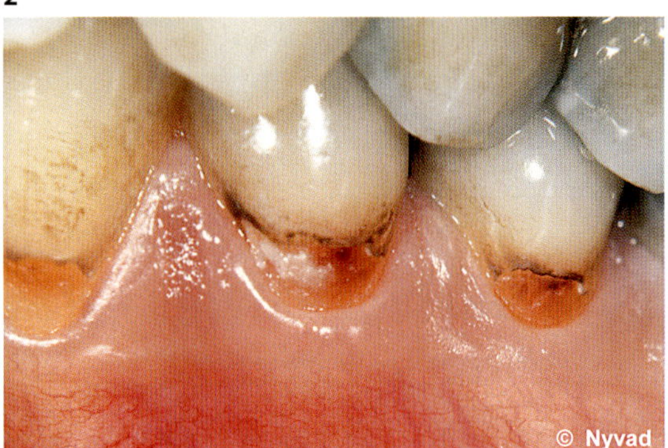

Fig. 1, 2. Non-cavitated (Fig. 1) and cavitated (Fig. 2) active root caries lesions. Note that lesions start at retention sites along the cemento-enamel junction and may spread along this structure or partly involve the cervical enamel. From Fejerskov and Nyvad [25], reproduced with permission.

3

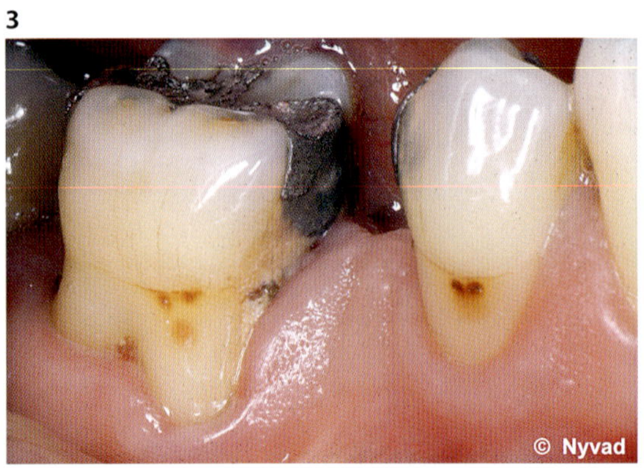

4

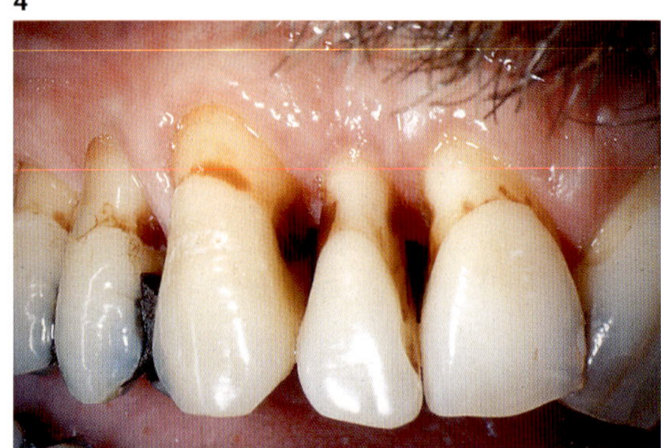

Fig. 3, 4. Small and narrow well-defined inactive root surface lesions. The lesions were arrested for a long period, as indicated by the clinically sound exposed root tissue gingival to the lesions. Fig. 3: From Fejerskov and Nyvad [25], reproduced with permission. Fig. 4: Courtesy of Ravald & Hamp [19].

particularly pronounced when root surfaces are regularly scaled and polished by dental health care professionals. Therefore, the clinical term root caries may include caries lesions in the cementum, but lesions occur mostly in the root dentin.

Diagnosing and choosing appropriate treatment for root surface caries requires basic knowledge of the clinical appearance and histopathology of the disease. These aspects are therefore discussed in detail in the following sections.

Clinical Features of Root Surface Caries

Root surface caries comprises a continuum of changes ranging from small, softened, and discolored spots on the root surface to extensive, brownish or very dark soft areas encircling the entire root surface (Fig. 1–4). Root caries lesions typically develop in "plaque stagnation areas" of the root, such as along the enamel-cementum junction, in surface irregularities, and along the gingival margin where the dental biofilm is more

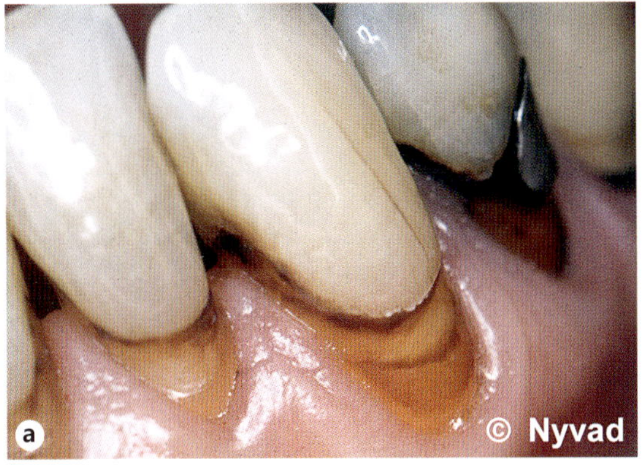

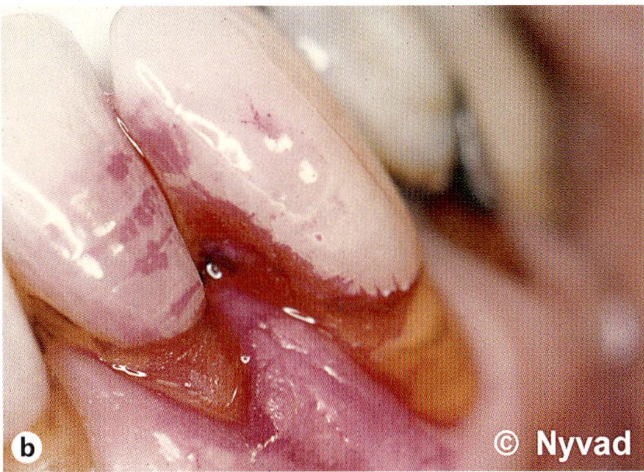

Fig. 5 a, b Biofilm formation in stagnation area. Removal of the biofilm reveals slowly progressing active root caries lesions along the cemento-enamel junction. Daily removal of this biofilm can arrest further lesion progression whereby the lesions turn into inactive lesions. From Fejerskov et al. [26], reproduced with permission.

difficult to remove during regular toothbrushing as seen in Figure 5a and b.

For purposes of treatment decisions, root caries lesions should be classified into "active" and "inactive" lesions. Active lesions are lesions that are considered to be progressing at the time of examination and hence need immediate professional treatment: non-operative or operative. Inactive lesions are considered to be arrested or slowly progressing, and further lesion progression may be controlled by daily toothbrushing with fluoride toothpaste, only.

Active lesions are yellowish or light brownish in color and are typically covered by a microbial deposit that may vary considerably in thickness (Fig. 1, 2). The carious tissue feels soft or leathery on gentle probing. There may be localized cavitation of the surface but soft areas of an active lesion may be extensive without obvious loss of tooth substance (Fig. 1). When cavitation occurs, the margins of the cavity are sharp and irregular (Fig. 2).

Lesions tend to spread laterally and often coalesce with minor neighboring lesions. The lesions may eventually encircle the tooth, in particular when they are located along the cemento-enamel junction (Fig. 4). It is of interest that the lesions rarely seem to extend in an apical direction as the gingival margin recedes. Rather new lesions develop at the recessed level of the gingival margin. This may occur irrespective of an inactive lesion being located more coronally.

The inactive (arrested) lesion is typically dark brown – often almost black (Fig. 3, 4). The surface of the lesion is usually shiny and smooth, and hard on gentle probing. This also applies when the lesion exhibits a frank cavity with distinct loss of tissue. However, if cavitation has occurred the margins most often appear smooth although the surface of the cavity is rough/uneven. In case of long-standing inactive lesions, the root surface may appear glossy and only discoloration suggests previous caries activity (Fig. 3).

In addition to these common types of lesions predominating in healthy individuals who perform regular oral hygiene, cases may occur in which almost the entire exposed root surface is covered by a layer of thick sticky biofilm (Fig. 6a). After the removal of the biofilm, the underlying darkly discolored leathery root surface may reveal minor macroscopic signs of cavitation (Fig. 6b). These types of slowly progressing lesions are predominantly observed in elderly patients showing

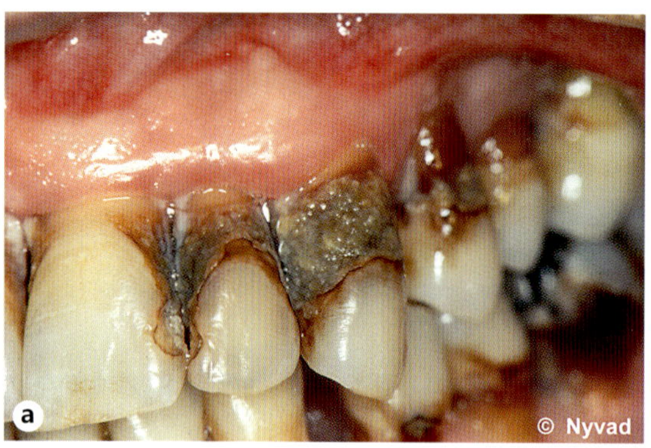

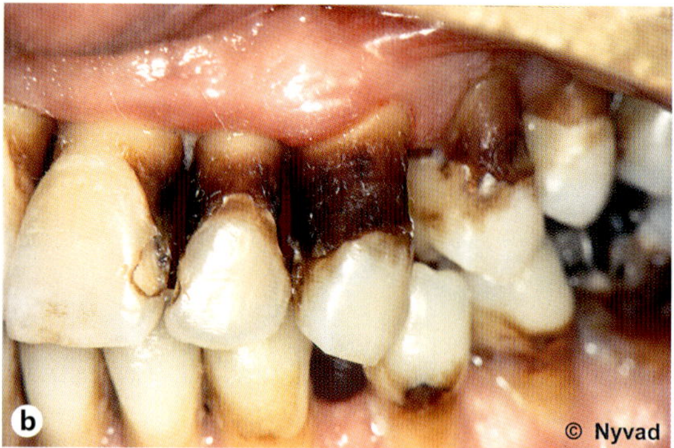

Fig. 6. a, b Root surfaces covered with extensive microbial biofilm. All surfaces exhibit widespread active root caries appearing dark and leathery on probing after the removal of the biofilm. Caries control applying daily meticulous oral hygiene and use of fluoridated toothpaste may be the only way to preserve the teeth as any attempt to perform traditional restorative treatment is likely to result in tooth fracture. From Fejerskov and Nyvad [25], reproduced with permission.

impaired salivary secretion due to medication or in patients who are unable to perform proper oral hygiene for various reasons.

This distinction between inactive and active stages of root surface caries is of clinical importance, as it shows that root surfaces react to the dynamic physicochemical processes taking place at the biofilm-root surface interface due to intermittent pH changes. If these processes are interfered by regular biofilm removal, active lesions may become arrested and converted to inactive lesions (see example in Figure 7a–d) [2]. Such a distinction is useful in recording the oral health status of the individual, as it gives an immediate impression of previous caries challenges as well as an indication of the need for active professional intervention and caries control at the time of examination.

Table 1 presents a summary of the recommended criteria to be used for differentiation between active and inactive root caries lesions. These criteria are typical characteristics of active and inactive root surface caries lesions. As emphasized before, caries lesions comprise a continuum of changes, and in the clinic some lesions may be difficult to classify definitively. It takes time to arrest an active root caries lesion (Fig. 7a–d). Moreover, inactive lesions may again convert into active lesions because of inadequate oral hygiene at that particular site. In our view, the term "inactive" covers lesions in which no further progression is expected to take place, provided there are no changes in caries risk factors, such as oral hygiene, diet, salivary flow, and medication. Nevertheless, minute areas within the surface of an inactive lesion may be covered by biofilm and demineralization may predominate at that particular spot. The classification, therefore, covers the lesion as a whole.

Histopathological Features of Root Surface Caries

To fully appreciate why it is important to differentiate lesions as active or inactive, it is crucial to understand the pathological changes taking place in the root dentin during lesion development.

Microradiographically, early root surface lesions appear as radiolucent zones in the outer part of the root surface (Fig. 8a–d). Even at the early stages, the lesions may extend into the dentin, although a relatively higher mineralized, 20- to 25-μm-thick, surface zone may be present [3,

Table 1. Clinical criteria for differentiating active and inactive root caries lesions

	Visual appearance	Tactile features
Active lesion	Yellowish or light brownish Dull/matte Typically covered by biofilm	Feels soft, sticky/leathery on gentle probing With/without localized/manifest cavitation Margins of cavity are sharply demarcated
Inactive lesion	Yellowish, brownish or black Shiny smooth Often not covered by biofilm	Feels hard on gentle probing Cavity formation may be rough/uneven Margins of cavity are smooth

4]. This hypermineralized surface zone is also a consistent finding in exposed root surfaces with no evidence of caries [5], whereas it is not present in non-exposed tissue [6, 7].

These observations indicate that the progressive loss of mineral from both enamel and root surfaces appears to follow similar physicochemical rules. They also imply that dissolved mineral may precipitate in the surface layer beneath the dental biofilm. Thus, exchange of mineral may be quite extensive at the cementum/dentin-biofilm fluid interface [5]. Furseth [8] has shown experimentally in vivo that topical treatment with fluoride may enhance this process of mineral deposition. Likewise , we have shown in experimental in situ studies how professional topical fluoride treatment combined with daily brushing with fluoride toothpaste helps to control root caries lesion progression, along with mineral uptake in the surface layer (Fig. 9, 10) [9]. These facts should be kept in mind when considering the relative importance of topical fluoride in the treatment of root surface caries at different stages of development; for review, see [1].

At the early stages of caries development in dental cementum, changes have been observed in hydroxyapatite crystals, and the exposed collagen fibers appear split [10, 11]. Furthermore, bacteria penetrate into cementum at an earlier stage in root surface caries than in coronal caries (Fig. 8a, d). Bacterial invasion takes place along the collagen fibers [11, 12] and may partly be responsible for the splitting of fibers.

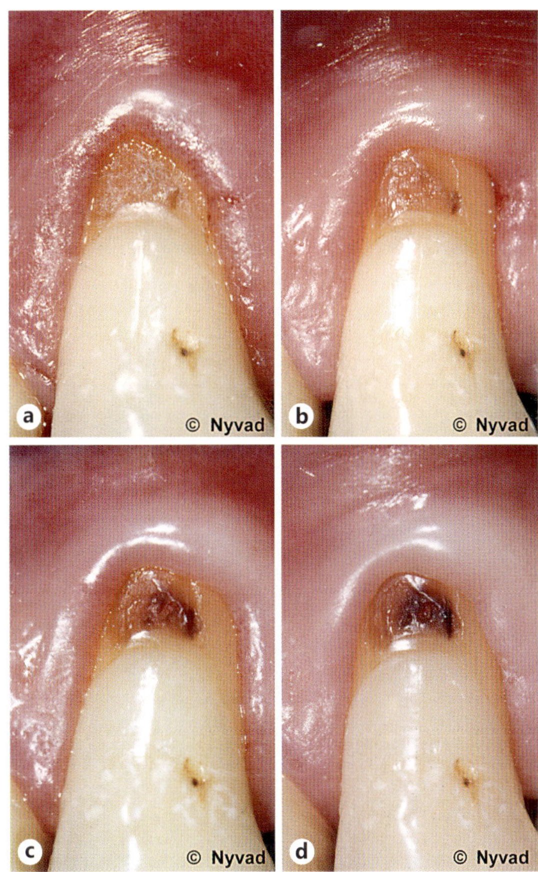

Fig. 7. a–d Successive stages of non-operative treatment of active root caries lesion on the buccal surface of upper left canine. The figure shows changes in the clinical appearance of the lesion after 3, 6, and 18 months (**b–d**), respectively. Note that improved oral hygiene leads to changes in color and surface structure of the lesion, from soft and yellowish to hard and darkly discolored. Also, note changes in the topography of the marginal gingiva. From Nyvad and Fejerskov [2], reproduced with permission.

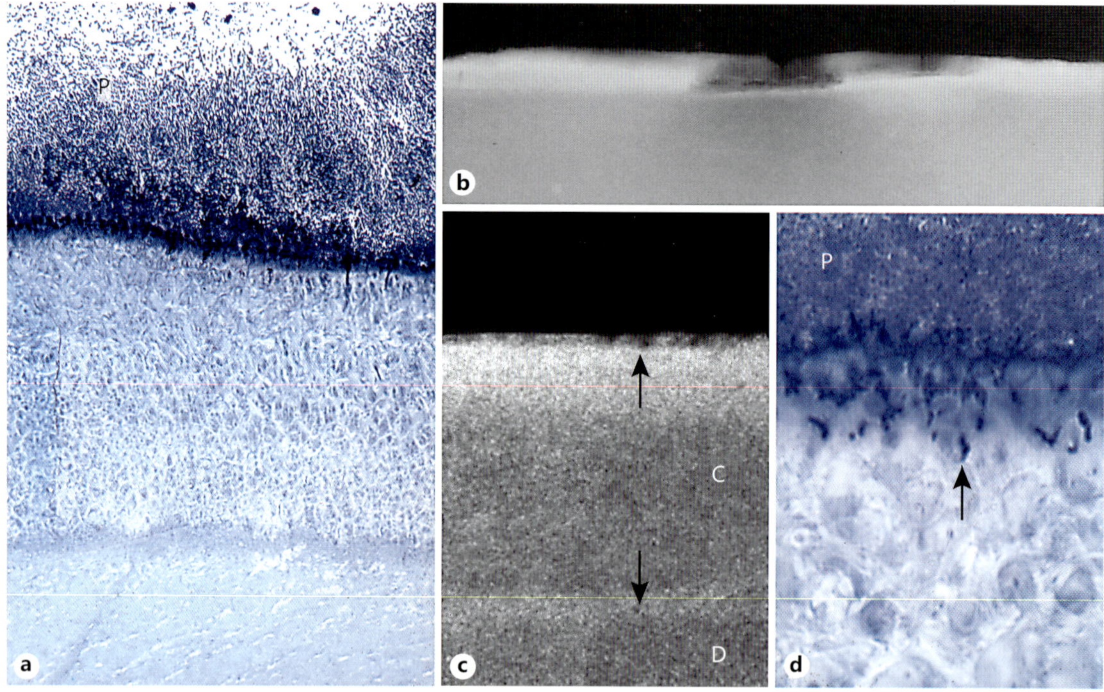

Fig. 8. a–d Two histological sections stained with toluidine blue and 2 microradiograms demonstrating early stages of root caries development. **a** Thin section with overview of root caries lesion covered by thick microbial deposits (P). **b** Microradiogram of subsurface lesion in cementum (radiopaque areas). **c**, **d** The surface layer of the lesion is invaded by bacteria at an early stage of the carious processes (see arrow in **d**). Thickness of the cementum is marked by 2 arrows in **c**. C, cementum, D, dentin. From Fejerskov and Nyvad [25], reproduced with permission.

At slightly more advanced stages of destruction (Fig. 11), the demineralization spreads into the underlying dentin, often extending several hundred microns below the surface. When shallow microcavities are observed, it is remarkable that even exposed dentinal surfaces may exhibit a relatively well-mineralized surface layer below which the demineralization occurs. In cases of localized breakdown of the dental cementum, bacteria invade the tissue along the incremental lines (Fig. 12).

Individual microcavities are often separated by areas of intact cementum that appear normal (Fig. 13). Such cavities are barely visible clinically or may develop into shallow clinically detectable cavities (Fig. 14). However, although the caries lesions may appear rather extensive, the lesions seldom extend more than 0.5–1 mm in depth [13, 14]. These observations are partly confirmed by histological observations by Westbrook et al. [15] who found that in 70% out of 140 lesions, the dentin had been invaded by microorganisms along with destruction of the dentinal matrix. However, they did not report on any changes in the dental pulp. These are pertinent findings that need to be confirmed as a slow rate of bacterial invasion and tissue degradation may significantly influence the choice of treatment of root surface caries. The number of dentinal tubules in root dentin is significantly smaller than in coronal dentin. In addition, a distinct hypermineralization (sclerosis) takes place in the root dentin with age. These features may partly explain why root surface caries progresses slowly. Finally, the microbial biofilm may be thinner and allow for

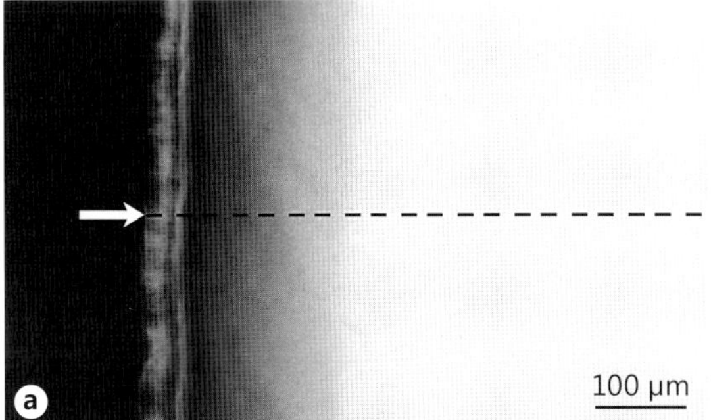

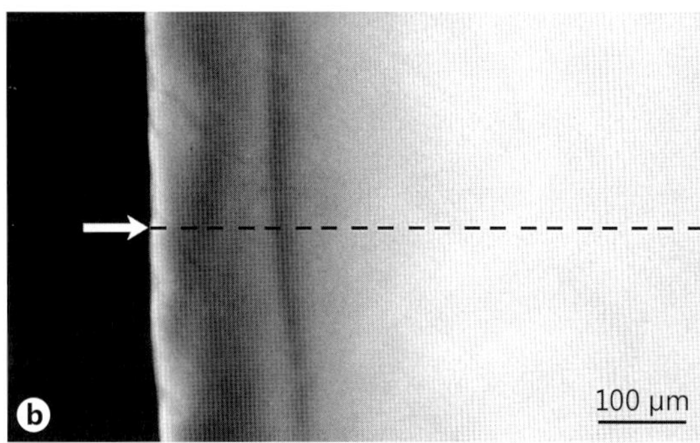

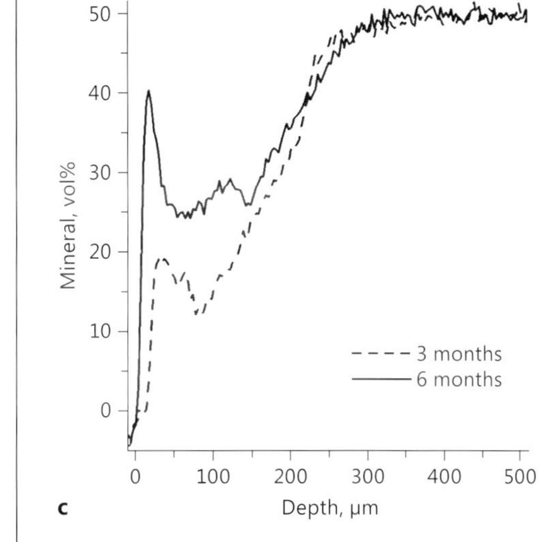

Fig. 9. a–c Micrographs of an experimental root caries lesion in situ. After 3 months (**a**), followed by 3 months (**b**) with daily biofilm removal and topical fluoride treatment. **c** The mineral content as a function of depth corresponding to the dotted lines in (**a**) and (**b**). The treatment resulted in an overall mineral gain because of an increase of the mineral content in the surface layer and formation of a zone of higher mineral content in the body of the lesion 125 µm deep to the surface. Scale bar = 100 µm. From Nyvad et al. [9], reproduced with permission.

better access to saliva, thereby enhancing the slow redeposition of minerals, which further slows down the progression of lesions.

The dentinal reactions to a caries challenge are indistinguishable from that reported for coronal caries, and there are thus very good biological explanations [16] for why root surface caries in general progresses relatively slowly as long as the individual has a normal salivary flow. Even when the root surface has been severely demineralized, the collagen fibers of the tissue are retained as a scaffold into which redeposition of mineral may take place. Great caution should, therefore, be taken to not remove or damage the softened tissue by probing, scaling, and polishing before any attempt to reharden the softened tissue through biofilm removal and topical fluoride treatment has been tried. Enabling mineral deposition into a partly demineralized root surface takes several months. The important factor is to ensure that the patient can perform a proper daily oral hygiene using a fluoridated toothpaste. Furthermore, a topical application of a 2% NaF solution or fluoride varnish is recommend at 3-month intervals as long as lesions show signs of activity.

Clinical Considerations and Implications

Several decades ago, caries progression in industrialized countries was so dramatic that it was common to consider restorative treatment as the

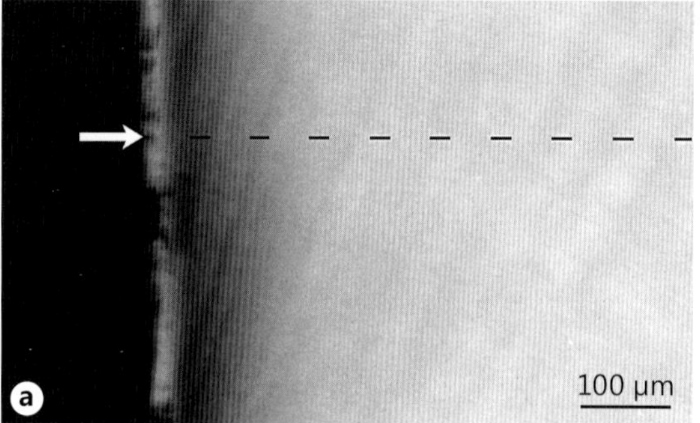

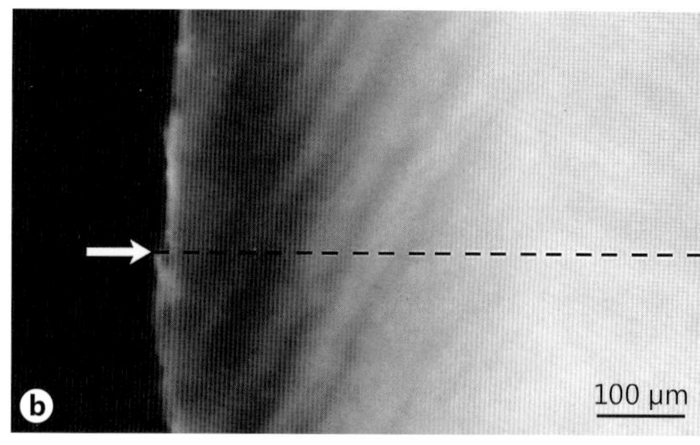

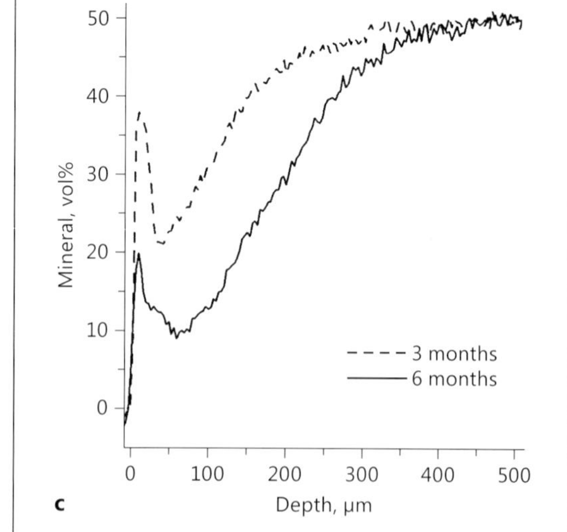

Fig. 10. a–c Micrographs of an experimental root caries lesion in situ. After 3 months (**a**) and 6 months (**b**) without daily biofilm removal. **c** The mineral content as a function of depth corresponding to the dotted lines in (**a**) and (**b**). Note that the lesion depth increased and the mineral content in the surface layer decreased over time. Scale bar = 100 μm. From Nyvad et al. [9], reproduced with permission.

treatment of choice to prevent further breakdown of the tissue and to restore the tooth ad integrum. However, increased knowledge of the dynamic processes involved in caries development suggests that active caries lesions can be transformed into arrested inactive lesions. These principles apply to dental enamel and to root surface caries (Fig. 7a–d). In favorable situations when the root surface is easily accessible to toothbrushing, even lesions with a distinct cavity extending rather deep into the dentin can be controlled and transformed into an inactive lesion [17]. Lesion arrest is facilitated by the combined effect of abrasion and a certain redeposition of mineral in the surface layer. It is, therefore, important as part of any treatment to decide whether the patient can perform adequate daily oral hygiene at the surfaces affected by active lesions.

Changing the environmental conditions does not only modify the surface features of the root caries lesions, but also enhances the biological response in the dentin, leading to increased sclerosis deep into the previously demineralized zone. These interventions may therefore have an effect on the experience of pain within weeks.

Proper oral hygiene is critical in caries control. No strict correlation has been found between oral hygiene status and root surface caries [18, 19]. However, the indices commonly used for quantifying oral hygiene do not take into account the quality of plaque removal in difficult-to-reach root surfaces. Lindhe and Nyman [20] showed that frequent

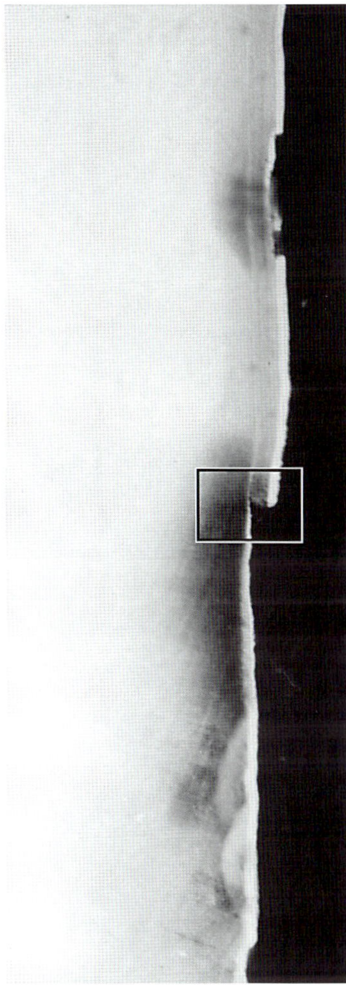

Fig. 11. Microradiogram of a root surface with several caries lesions separated from each other by unaffected areas. Note how the cementum layers are lost during caries lesion progression. The lesions show a subsurface type of demineralization with the surface layer containing a high mineral content. From Fejerskov and Nyvad [25], reproduced with permission.

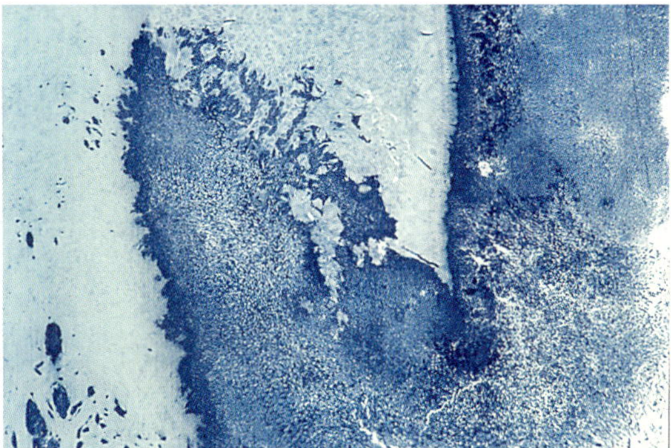

Fig. 12. The histological section originates from the upper border of the larger lesion in Figure 11 (see frame). Note how bacteria invade the cementum and the underlying dentin. From Fejerskov and Nyvad [25], reproduced with permission.

plaque removal by professionals in conjunction with daily use of fluoride toothpaste almost totally prevents root surface caries development. These observations concur with the conclusions of DePaola et aI. [21], who inferred in a study on clinical factors associated with root surface caries that "the common factor underlying most if not all of the subgroup differences is oral hygiene, which must therefore be a major disease determinant."

It may be impossible to institute this type of thorough caries control for all patients with exposed root surfaces. It is, therefore, important to identify patients at higher risk of developing root surface caries. Despite a very extensive preventive program, periodontally treated patients developed new caries lesions on 5% of the exposed root surfaces in a study in Sweden [19]. Half of the patients experienced new root surface lesions during the 4 years of observation. These individuals could have been identified at the initial examination by their previous root surface caries experience!!

The basic histological similarity between coronal and root surface caries (despite distinct differences in the structural composition of the tissues) indicates that very similar physicochemical processes are responsible for caries development and progression in the 2 tissues. It is, therefore, expected that topical fluorides play an important role in controlling caries processes by slowing down the rate of lesion progression [22]. In situ studies by Nyvad et al. [9] (Fig. 9, 10) provided convincing evidence that fluoride is essential in root caries control. A recent systematic review concluded that root caries control strategies

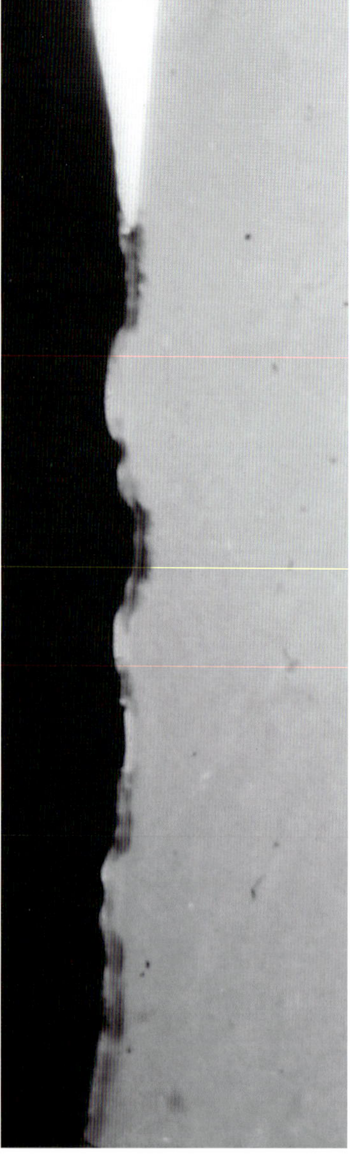

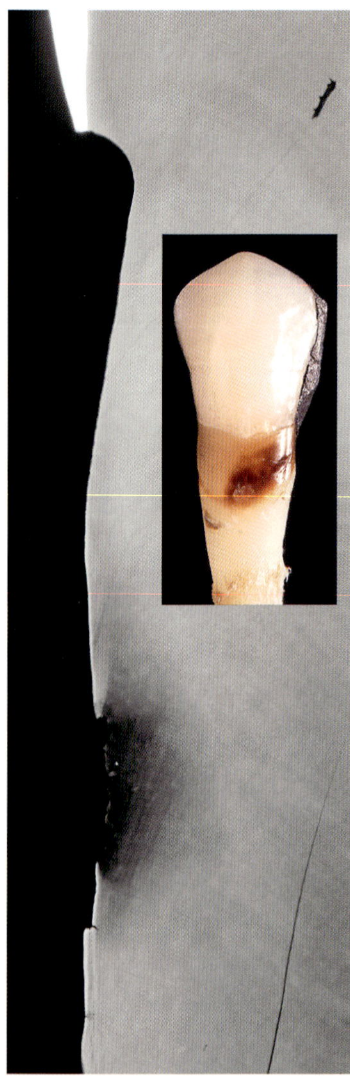

Fig. 13. Microradiogram illustrating several shallow caries lesions mainly confined to the cementum, with a typical subsurface demineralization. From Fejerskov and Nyvad [25], reproduced with permission.
Fig. 14. The macroscopical picture (**inset**) shows an extracted tooth with a dark inactive lesion. The surface is shiny except for the small cavity in the lower part of the lesion. The microradiogram suggests that the shiny surface developed as a result of abrasion due to toothbrushing. However, a localized cavity with distinct surface loss and sharply demarcated borders extends into dentin. From Nyvad and Fejerskov [4], reproduced with permission.

should embrace a non-operative approach with daily brushing with fluoride toothpaste. Active decay might be inactivated if improved oral hygiene is combined with professional application of fluoride varnishes/solutions or self-applied toothpastes containing high fluoride concentrations [1]. Needless to say, the professional fluoride application should always be accompanied by meticulous oral hygiene and sugar control to optimize the caries-controlling effect.

The consequences of this knowledge are essential when considering whether a root caries lesion needs restoration by a filling or attempts should aim at arresting active lesions. If thorough professional tooth cleaning is combined with fluoride treatment, as in the patient shown in Figure 15 even extensive active root surface lesions can be rehardened. Although the lesions may extend over a large area, they are usually shallow. As emphasized before, lesions inevitably become brownish or black in color, characteristic of inactive lesions. There may even be frank cavitations. Nevertheless, if the patient can accept this cosmetic appearance, even a black, concave but hard area on the root surface is better than a deteriorating restoration that is difficult to keep clean, and with caries inevitably developing along the faulty margins. Then, by combining the knowledge of the dynamics of the caries process and the benefits of the tissue responses in the pulpo-dentinal organ, numerous fillings may be avoided in elderly patients.

If, however, root lesions have reached a depth at which the performance of proper oral hygiene is difficult, operative caries treatment is required. Despite improvements in filling materials, treatment of root caries is still very difficult. Only 65% of root caries lesions restored with glass-ionomer cement in elderly patients survived after 2 years [23]. No studies have evaluated the longevity of root caries restorations for more than 2 years. Irrespective of the restorative material applied (glass ionomer or composite resin), the majority of fillings may fail because of dislodgement, possibly because of difficulties in achieving moisture control [24]. The poor prognosis of operative treatment of root surface caries indicates that operative treatment should be avoided as far as possible in favor of non-operative caries control strategies.

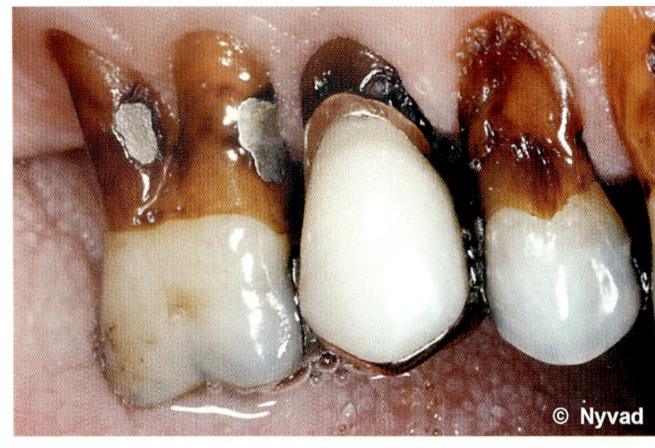

Fig. 15. Inactive root caries lesions with hard and shiny surfaces despite the brownish color. This result of a successful caries control demonstrates why it is not recommended to start traditional restorative treatment for patients who master regular careful biofilm control. From Fejerskov and Nyvad [25], reproduced with permission.

Conclusion

If today's knowledge of etiology and pathogenesis of dental caries is combined with the modern concepts on cariostatic mechanisms of fluorides, it is apparent that root surface caries can be controlled by very simple means: daily oral hygiene using a fluoride containing toothpaste combined with restriction of the intake of sugars (snacks, soft drinks, sweets, and so on). Because operative treatment has a very poor prognosis on root surfaces, a proper clinical diagnosis and non-operative caries control strategies are mandatory!

References

1 Heasman PA, Ritchie M, Asuni A, Gavillet E, Simonsen JL, Nyvad B: Gingival recession and root caries in the ageing population: a critical evaluation of treatments. J Clin Periodontol 2017;44(suppl 18):S178–S193.

2 Nyvad B, Fejerskov O: Active root surface caries converted into inactive caries as a response to oral hygiene. Scand J Dent Res 1986;94:281–284.

3 Furseth R, Johansen E: A microradiographic comparison of sound and carious human dental cementum. Arch Oral Biol 1968;13:1197–1206.

4 Nyvad B, Fejerskov O: Active and inactive root surface caries – structural entities?; in Thylstrup A, Leach SA, Qvist V (eds): Dentine and Dentine Reactions in the Oral Cavity. Oxford, IRL Press, 1987, pp 165–179.

5 Selvig KA: Biological changes at the tooth-saliva interface in periodontal disease. J Dent Res 1969;48:846–855.

6 Hals E, Selvig KA: Correlated electron probe microanalysis and microradiography of carious and normal dental cementum. Caries Res 1977;11:62–75.

7 Tohda H, Fejerskov O, Yanagisawa T: Transmission electron microscopy of cementum crystals correlated with Ca and F distribution in normal and carious human root surfaces. J Dent Res 1996;75:949–954.
8 Furseth R: A study of experimentally exposed and fluoride treated dental cementum in pigs. Acta Odontol Scand 1970;28:833–850.
9 Nyvad B, ten Cate JM, Fejerskov O: Arrest of root surface caries in situ. J Dent Res 1997;76:1845–1853.
10 Schüpbach P, Guggenheim B, Lutz F: Human root caries: histopathology of initial lesions in cementum and dentin. J Oral Pathol Med 1989;18:146–156.
11 Nyvad B, Fejerskov O: An ultrastructural study of bacterial invasion and tissue breakdown in human experimental root-surface caries. J Dent Res 1990;69: 1118–1125.
12 Frank RM, Steuer P, Hemmerle J: Ultrastructural study on human root caries. Caries Res 1989;12:209–217.
13 Sumney DL, Jordan HV, Englander HR: The prevalence of root surface caries in selected population. J Periodontol 1973; 44:500–504.
14 Banting DW, Courtright PN: Distribution and natural history of carious lesions on the roots of teeth. Dent J 1975; 41:45–49.
15 Westbrook JL, Miller AS, Chilton NW, Williams FL, Mumma RD Jr: Root surface caries: a clinical, histopathologic and microradiographic investigation. Caries Res 1974;8:249–255.
16 Fejerskov O: Pathology of dental caries; in Fejerskov O, Nyvad B, Kidd EA (eds): Dental Caries: The Disease and Its Clinical Management, ed 3. Oxford, Whiley Blackwell, 2015, pp 40–81.
17 Nyvad B, Fejerskov O: Assessing the stage of caries lesion activity on the basis of clinical and microbiological examination. Community Dent Oral Epidemiol 1997;25:69–75.
18 Hix JO, O'leary TJ: The relationship between cemental caries, oral hygiene status and fermentable carbohydrate intake. J Periodontol 1979;47:398–404.
19 Ravald N, Hamp SE: Prediction of root surface caries in patients treated for advanced periodontal disease. J Clin Periodontol 1981;8:400–414.
20 Lindhe J, Nyman S: The effect of plaque control and surgical pocket elimination on the establishment and maintenance of periodontal health. A longitudinal study of periodontal therapy in cases of advanced disease. J Clin Periodontol 1975;2:67–79.
21 DePaola PF, Soparkar PM, Tavares M, Kent RL Jr: Clinical profiles of individuals with and without root surface caries. Gerodontology 1989;8:9–15.
22 Fejerskov O, Thylstrup A, Larsen MJ: Rational use of fluorides in caries prevention. A concept based on possible cariostatic mechanisms. Acta Odontol Scand 1981;39:241–249.
23 Hu JY, Chen XC, Li YQ, Smales RJ, Yip KH: Radiation-induced root surface caries restored with glass-ionomer cement placed in conventional and ART cavity preparations: results at two years. Aust Dent J 2005;50:186–190.
24 Levy SM, Jensen ME: A clinical evaluation of the restoration of root surface caries. Spec Care Dentist 1990;10:156–160.
25 Fejerskov O, Nyvad B: Pathology and treatment of dental caries in the ageing individual; in Holm-Petersen P, Löe H (eds): Geriatric Dentistry. Copenhagen, Munksgaard, 1986, pp 238–262.
26 Fejerskov O, Nyvad B, Kidd EAM: Clinical appearances of caries lesions; in Fejerskov O, Kidd E (eds): Dental Caries. Oxford, Blackwell Munksgaard, 2008, pp 7–18.

Prof. Bente Nyvad
Department of Dentistry and Oral Health, Aarhus University
Vennelyst Boulevard 9
DK–8000 Aarhus C (Denmark)
E-Mail Nyvad@odont.au.dk

Carrilho MRO (ed): Root Caries: From Prevalence to Therapy.
Monogr Oral Sci. Basel, Karger, 2017, vol 26, pp 55–62 (DOI: 10.1159/000479343)

Assessing the Risk of Developing Carious Lesions in Root Surfaces

Sophie Doméjean[a] • Avijit Banerjee[b]

[a]Université Clermont Auvergne, UFR d'Odontologie, CHU Clermont-Ferrand, Service d'Odontologie, Clermont-Ferrand, France; [b]Chair/Head of Department, Conservative & MI Dentistry, King's College London Dental Institute at Guy's Hospital, King's Health Partners, London, UK

Abstract

Patients' susceptibility to coronal and root caries (RC) is modulated by a range of biological, environmental, social, psychological, and behavior-related factors. These factors, considered either in isolation or combined into specific models, contribute to the overall patient susceptibility/risk of new lesion occurrence and/or of existing lesion progression, allowing the oral healthcare team to define specific and individualized preventive and curative regimens. Various caries susceptibility/risk assessment (CRA) protocols/models have been developed to assist the oral healthcare practitioner/team in a logical systematic approach to synthesize information about the caries disease process with its multifactorial etiology. These protocols/models consider caries susceptibility/risk in general without any specific localization of the caries process; none of them specifically consider the risk of developing carious lesions in root surfaces. This chapter aims to discuss CRA related to RC lesions in terms of prediction of both the occurrence of new RC lesions and of continuing progression of existing lesions.

Introduction

Minimal intervention (MI) oral healthcare is now becoming the proven, ethical rationale for the appropriate management of oral/dental disease and maintenance of health and patient wellbeing. Patient-focused, team-delivered MI oral healthcare provision should not be planned at the lesion level but at the patient level, depending on their needs whilst managing expectations and outcomes [1–10]. The management of root caries (RC) is not any different.

RC susceptibility/risk is multifactorial and involves variations in the oral environment, periodontal status, invading microorganisms in sub-gingival plaque, and host-derived proteolytic enzymes contained in saliva, gingival crevicular fluid, and dentin itself [11]. Like coronal carious lesions, RC lesions are preventable and, if diagnosed and managed early in the caries process, they have the potential to remineralize without the need for surgical, operative inter-

Table 1. CRA systems and their target populations

Systems/protocols (classified by alphabetic order)	Target populations		Root exposure taken into account
	infants and children under 6	children aged 6 years and over, adolescents, and adults	
ADA system [21, 30]	√	√	√*
CAMBRA system [20, 27, 28]	√	√	√*
Caries risk pyramid [29]		√	
Cariogram [26]		√	
CAT of the AAPD [23]	√	√	
DCRAM [22]	√		
ICCMS™ caries risk-likelihood matrix [49, 50]	√	√	
MySmileBuddy [24, 25]	√		

None of the CRA systems are specific to RC prediction assessment; only the Cariogram has been tested for RC prediction [32]. AAPD, American Academy of Pediatric Dentistry; ADA, American Dental Association; CAMBRA, caries management by risk assessment; CAT, Caries Assessment Tool; DCRAM, Dundee Caries Risk Assessment Model; ICCMS™, International Caries Classification and Management System™.
* Only taken into account for patients aged over 6 years old and/or adults.

vention [12–15]. Thus, the ability to assess a patient's RC susceptibility to developing root surface carious lesions accurately is crucial for the determination and implementation of appropriate patient-focused preventive strategies, leading to the reduced need for complex operative treatments and associated morbidity [16].

This chapter aims to discuss the caries susceptibility/risk assessment (CRA) related to RC lesions in terms of prediction of both the occurrence of new RC lesions and of continuing progression of existing lesions.

Are There Any CRA Systems/Protocols Specific to RC Development?

Coronal and RC susceptibilities are modulated by a range of biological, environmental, social, psychological, and behavior-related factors [15, 17, 18]. Various CRA protocols/models have been developed to assist the oral healthcare practitioners and their team in a logical systematic approach to synthesizing information about the caries disease process with its multifactorial etiology [19]. These can be divided into 2 groups according to the age of the patient, under [20–25] or over 6 years old [21, 23, 26–30] (Table 1). None of the cited systems/protocols are specifically related to RC. They all consider caries susceptibility/risk in general without any specific localization of the caries process (coronal surfaces, root surfaces or caries adjacent to restorations and sealants (formerly known as secondary/recurrent carious lesions)). Thus, none of the cited CRA systems/protocols consider specifically the risk of developing carious lesions in root surfaces per se. This may not have much clinical relevance in infants, children, and adolescents where root surfaces are rarely exposed and CRA of RC is not a matter of clinical importance. However, in adults and the older population, the lack of such susceptibility assessment may be deemed a problem, especially in the light of the latest data related to the RC prevalence (see the second chapter by Hayes et al., this volume, pp. 9–14). Only 2 of the cited systems/protocols, CAMBRA [28] and ADA [21], take the item "exposed roots" into account but not in order to assess the risk of RC development itself but to assess the overall patient susceptibility to develop carious lesions in general (whatever the surface). Bauer et al. [31] developed a model to pattern RC development and predict RC progression in older adults (over 65 years) over 18-month cycles. The model is valid for 2 cycles, totaling 36 months and shows that a sound root surface has a high probability to remain caries-free and that on the contrary, one- and 2-surface lesions aggressively affect other adjoining surfaces. The model showed that maintaining sound root surfaces reduces the risk of tooth dysfunction (morphological destruction) and loss and that, once a lesion is present, early treatment intervention is indicated to reduce the need for more complicated and expensive dental services and to prevent tooth loss. This data weighs in favor of the importance of MI based on primary, secondary, and tertiary preventions but does not help the practitioner to target the individualized factors and develop a personalized oral healthcare plan with the patient.

Cariogram, originally developed for general caries susceptibility assessment, has been tested for its performance in predicting RC incidence over a 24-month period, among 280 patients aged over 65 years [32]. The results showed that Cariogram may be useful clinically in determining future RC risk in independently living older adults. Indeed, the mean RC increment was higher in the group identified at baseline as being at higher risk compared to the lowest risk group. A significantly higher mean RC increment was observed in patients with frequent dietary sugar intake, poorer plaque control, those avoiding fluoride use, and xerostomic individuals. Moreover, a minimized Cariogram model, without inclusion of any salivary variables, also showed a predictive ability for RC, which did not differ significantly from that of the comprehensive model.

What Are the Factors Related to RC Development?

A systematic review (2010) [33] examined 2 key questions: can RC incidence be predicted by risk models based on subject characteristics and if so, which risk indicators are associated consistently and strongly with RC incidence? It included data extracted from articles published between 1970 and June 2009, which reported information on RC incidence, risk indicators, and/or regression models. Variables most frequently tested and significantly associated with RC incidence were baseline RC incidence, number of teeth, and plaque index. It showed a substantial variation between the 13 selected articles related to RC risk models in terms of methodology (variable selection, sample size, outcome assessment methods, incidence periods, and so on) limiting the applicability of findings to guide targeted clinical prevention regimens. As mentioned above, there is a lack of integrated systems/protocols specifically assessing the risk of carious lesion development on root surfaces.

Nevertheless, since the publication of this systematic review, other studies investigated the factors associated with RC experience as shown in Table 2. Table 2 shows the variability among studies in terms of populations (e.g., countries, number of patients, age groups, and so on). Among the 15 references listed, only 3 are related to prospective studies [32, 34, 35] whilst the others are observational cross-sectional surveys [36–47]. Three observational cross-sectional studies [39, 40, 42] compared 2 different age groups of patients 35–44 [39, 40] and 45–64 years old [42] with patients aged over 65 years and older. They showed that RC experience was different (increased RC prevalence in the older groups) among the examined groups, illustrating that caries prevention programs should address relevant age-based risk factors.

Table 3 summarizes the factors that are significantly related to RC incidence (in prospective

Table 2. Surveys assessing prediction models or factors associated with RC published since Ritter et al. [33] systematic review, (references are classified by chronological and alphabetic order)

References	Populations	Country	Type of study
Sugihara et al. [36], 2010	153 elderly patients 60–94 years old; mean age 73.5 years Relatively healthy elderly who did not need any special care in their daily lives	Japan	Observational cross-sectional study
Sánchez-García et al. [35], 2011	531 patients Over 60 years old; mean age 71.8 years	Mexico	Prospective study over 12 months
Ellefsen et al. [37], 2012	61 patients with recent diagnosis of Alzheimer's disease 70–95 years old; mean age 82.8 years	Denmark	Observational cross-sectional study
Islas-Granillo et al. [38], 2012	85 patients living in long-term care facilities, or independently and attending an elder day-care group 60 years and older; mean age 78 years	Mexico	Observational cross-sectional study
Mamai-Homata et al. [39], 2012	1,188 patients; 35–44 years old 1,093 patients; 65–74 years old	Greece	Observational cross-sectional study Comparison: 2 age groups: 35–44 and 65–74
Gökalp and and Doğan, [40], 2012	1,631 patients; 35–44 years old 1,545 patients; 65–74 years old	Turkey	Observational cross-sectional study Comparison: 2 age groups: 35–44 and 65–74
Ritter et al. [41], 2012	437 patients; 21–80 years old	USA	Observational cross-sectional study
Chi et al. [42], 2013	775 patients; 45–97 years old; mean age 63.2 years	USA	Observational cross-sectional study Comparison: 45–64 years old and older
Tan et al. [43], 2014	306 non-frail elders living in residential homes At least 5 teeth with exposed roots 62–92 years old; mean age 78.8 years	Hong Kong	Observational cross-sectional study
Hayes et al. [44], 2016	334 independently living older adults with basic self-care ability Mean age 69.1; median age 68 years	Ireland	Observational cross-sectional study
Kumara-Raja et al. [45], 2016	312 patients living at residential homes 60 years and older; mean age 71 years	India	Observational cross-sectional study
Ritter et al. [34], 2016	301 caries-active adult patients	USA	Prospective study over 3 years
D'Avila et al. [46], 2017	785 patients living independently 60 years and older; mean age 66.9 years	Brazil	Observational cross-sectional study
Hariyani et al. [47], 2017	5,505 patients 15–91 years old; mean age 50 years	Australia	Observational cross-sectional study
Hayes et al. [32], 2017	280 patients living independently Aged over 65 years	Ireland	Prospective study over 2 years Cariogram evaluation

Table 3. Factors associated with RC in elderly patients in the publications since Ritter et al.'s [33] systematic review (classified by alphabetic order)

Investigated factors	Studies in which the factor is significantly associated with RC		
	prospective studies	cross-sectional studies isolated factors	cross-sectional studies multifactorial analyses and models
Age		[37, 39–42, 47]	[46]
Coronal carious lesions		[37]	[44]
Dental attendance patterns		[40, 41]	
Denture wear/contact		[36, 43]	
Depressive symptoms		[46]	
Diet	[32]	[45]	
Dry mouth/xerostomia/low stimulated saliva flow	[32]		[36, 43, 45]
Education level		[38, 39]	
Ethnicity	[34]	[41]	
Exposed roots/gingival recessions		[36, 43]	[36, 44]
Filled or decayed root surfaces/RC index	[34, 35]	[37, 42]	
Gender	[34]	[41, 45]	[46]
Healthy root surfaces	[35]		
Increased number of root surfaces at risk	[34]		
Limitations in basic daily life activities	[35]		
Lower income/socioeconomic status		[45, 47]	
Marital status (being single)		[38, 45]	
Medications		[45]	
Mutans streptococci level	[35]		
No fluoride use	[32]		
No mouthwash use	[35]		
No toothbrushing		[38–40, 45, 47]	[46]
Number of follow-up years at risk	[34]		
Number of teeth			[36]
Periodontal disease/bleeding on probing		[36]	[36]
Poor plaque control	[32]	[38, 43, 47]	[44]
Poor self-reported oral health		[41]	
Publicly funded long-term care		[38]	
RC at baseline	[34]		
Recent professional fluoride treatment		[41]	
Rural residence		[39, 40]	[46]
Smoking	[34, 35]	[47]	[36]
Upper anterior region		[43]	

In bold letters: factors that were described like being associated to RC experience by Ritter et al. [33].

studies) or RC experience (in cross-sectional studies using univariate and/or multivariate analyses). The multiplicity and the variability of factors taken into account among studies show the real complexity of RC susceptibility assessment.

Table 4 lists a set of factors extracted from Table 3 that could be combined for RC risk assessment in older patients. They do not differ dramatically from those included, for example, in the CAMBRA system. Nevertheless, specific at-

Table 4. Suggestion of classification of factors that have been shown to be significantly associated with RC in recent observational cross-sectional and prospective studies

Classification of factors associated with RC experience	
Socio-demographic characteristics	Age Gender Ethnicity Socioeconomic status (education, income) Marital status Residence: rural/urban; living independently/long-term care Dental attendance patterns
General health	Depressive symptoms Medications Limitations in basic daily life activities Smoking habits
Oral status and caries experience (on both coronal and root surfaces)	Poor self-reported oral health Number of teeth Coronal carious lesions RC experience at baseline (filled/decayed root surfaces) Exposed roots/gingival recessions Denture (wear/contact) Dry mouth/xerostomia Mutans Streptococci level
Oral hygiene	Poor plaque control Toothbrushing habits Fluoride use Mouthwash use

tention should be drawn to factors related to more advanced ages, such as exposed roots, RC experience, way of living (independent or not), and limitations in basic daily lifestyle-related activities.

RC Management in Oral Healthcare Practice

Very little is known about how oral healthcare practitioners and their teams deal with RC in everyday practice, and to our knowledge, a unique survey on the topic has been undertaken by Garton and Ford using a questionnaire to describe how Queensland dental practitioners perceived the issue of RC in terms of occurrence, predisposing factors, diagnosis, and management [48]. The respondents demonstrated an awareness of RC despite a lack of consistency with respect to risk assessment strategies. They showed that the majority of respondents (77%) reported not recording RC in a way that could be distinguished from coronal lesions. They perceived that they encounter RC most often in patients aged 55 years and over. Dietary analysis was the most commonly reported adjunctive aid for risk assessment. Salivary impairment was reported to be an important risk factor for RC by 93% of respondents, but only 18% reported performing salivary analysis.

Further research in the area is necessary to understand factors dentists use to derive general caries risk/susceptibility scores for their patients [42].

Conclusions

RC is a preventable non-communicable disease that affects a growing number of adults, especially the elderly. Prevention could be targeted and optimized if high-risk individuals could be identified. This study shows that certain factors are related to RC experience, but that there is a lack of any specific model/system to assess the risk of developing carious lesions in root surfaces. Indeed the specific contribution of each of the factors recognized to influence RC experience of an individual or within a population has yet to be investigated in multicenter prospective studies of potentially high-risk populations. Moreover, further surveys in different clinical settings must investigate the professional oral healthcare practices related to RC management.

References

1 Dawson AS, Makinson OF: Dental treatment and dental health. Part 1. A review of studies in support of a philosophy of Minimum Intervention Dentistry. Aust Dent J 1992;37:126–132.
2 Dawson AS, Makinson OF: Dental treatment and dental health. Part 2. An alternative philosophy and some new treatment modalities in operative dentistry. Aust Dent J 1992;37:205–210.
3 Sheiham A: Minimal intervention in dental care. Med Princ Pract 2002; 11(suppl 1):2–6.
4 Bowley J: Minimal intervention prosthodontics: current knowledge and societal implications. Med Princ Pract 2002; 11(suppl 1):22–31.
5 Elderton RJ: Preventive (evidence-based) approach to quality general dental care. Med Princ Pract 2003;12(suppl 1):12–21.
6 Featherstone JD, Doméjean S: Minimal intervention dentistry: part 1. From ‘compulsive’ restorative dentistry to rational therapeutic strategies. Br Dent J 2012;213:441–445.
7 Frencken JE, Peters MC, Manton DJ, Leal SC, Gordan VV, Eden E: Minimal intervention dentistry for managing dental caries – a review: report of a FDI task group. Int Dent J 2012;62:223–243.
8 Pitts NB, Zero DT, Marsh PD, Ekstrand K, Weintraub JA, Ramos-Gomez F, Tagami J, Twetman S, Tsakos G, Ismail A: Dental caries. Nat Rev Dis Primers 2017; 3:17030.
9 Banerjee A: 'MI'opia or 20/20 vision? Br Dent J 2013;214:101–105.
10 Banerjee A, Doméjean S: The contemporary approach to tooth preservation: minimum intervention (MI) caries management in general practice. Prim Dent J 2013;2:30–37.
11 Takahashi N, Nyvad B: Ecological hypothesis of dentin and root caries. Caries Res 2016;50:422–431.
12 Leake JL: Clinical decision-making for caries management in root surfaces. J Dent Educ 2001;65:1147–1153.
13 Fernández CE, Tenuta LMA, Del Bel Cury AA, Nóbrega DF, Cury JA: Effect of 5,000 ppm fluoride dentifrice or 1,100 ppm fluoride dentifrice combined with acidulated phosphate fluoride on caries lesion inhibition and repair. Caries Res 2017;51:179–187.
14 Wierichs RJ, Meyer-Lueckel H: Systematic review on noninvasive treatment of root caries lesions. J Dent Res 2015;94: 261–271.
15 Tinanoff N: Dental caries risk assessment and prevention. Dent Clin North Am 1995;39:709–719.
16 Garton BJ, Ford PJ: Root caries and diabetes: risk assessing to improve oral and systemic health outcomes. Aust Dent J 2012;57:114–122.
17 Featherstone JD: Prevention and reversal of dental caries: role of low level fluoride. Community Dent Oral Epidemiol 1999;27:31–40.
18 Featherstone JD: Dental caries: a dynamic disease process. Aust Dent J 2008; 53:286–291.
19 Doméjean S, Banerjee A, Featherstone JDB: Caries risk/susceptibility assessment: its value in minimum intervention oral healthcare. Br Dent J 2017;223: 191–197.
20 Ramos-Gomez FJ, Crall J, Gansky SA, Slayton RL, Featherstone JD: Caries risk assessment appropriate for the age 1 visit (infants and toddlers). J Calif Dent Assoc 2007;35:687–702.
21 American Dental Association (ADA): Caries risk assessment form (age 0–6). https://www.ada.org (accessed June 2017).
22 Macritchie HM, Longbottom C, Robertson M, Nugent Z, Chan K, Radford JR, Pitts NB: Development of the Dundee Caries Risk Assessment Model (DCRAM) – risk model development using a novel application of CHAID analysis. Community Dent Oral Epidemiol 2012;40:37–45.
23 American Academy of Pediatric Dentistry: Guideline on caries-risk assessment and management for infants, children, and adolescents. Pediatr Dent 2015;37:132–139.
24 Custodio-Lumsden CL, Wolf RL, Contento IR, Basch CE, Zybert PA, Koch PA, Edelstein BL: Validation of an early childhood caries risk assessment tool in a low-income Hispanic population. J Public Health Dent 2016;76:136–142.
25 Levine J, Wolf RL, Chinn C, Edelstein BL: MySmileBuddy: an iPad-based interactive program to assess dietary risk for early childhood caries. J Acad Nutr Diet 2012;112:1539–1542.
26 Bratthall D, Hänsel Petersson G: Cariogram – a multifactorial risk assessment model for a multifactorial disease. Community Dent Oral Epidemiol 2005;33: 256–264.

27 Featherstone JD, Adair SM, Anderson MH, Berkowitz RJ, Bird WF, Crall JJ, Den Besten PK, Donly KJ, Glassman P, Milgrom P, et al: Caries management by risk assessment: consensus statement, April 2002. J Calif Dent Assoc 2003;31: 257–269.
28 Featherstone JD, Domejean-Orliaguet S, Jenson L, Wolff M, Young DA: Caries risk assessment in practice for age 6 through adult. J Calif Dent Assoc 2007; 35:703–707, 710–713.
29 Morou-Bermúdez E, Billings RJ, Burne RA, Elías-Boneta A: Caries risk pyramid: a practical biological approach to caries management by risk assessment. P R Health Sci J 2011;30:165–166.
30 American Dental Association (ADA): Caries risk assessment form (age >6). https://www.ada.org (accessed June 2017).
31 Bauer JG, Spackman S, Dong J, Garrett N: Predictor model of root caries in older adults: reporting of evidence to the translational evidence mechanism. Open Dent J 2010;4:124–132.
32 Hayes M, Da Mata C, McKenna G, Burke FM, Allen PF: Evaluation of the Cariogram for root caries prediction. J Dent 2017;62:25–30.
33 Ritter AV, Shugars DA, Bader JD: Root caries risk indicators: a systematic review of risk models. Community Dent Oral Epidemiol 2010;38:383–397.
34 Ritter AV, Preisser JS, Puranik CP, Chung Y, Bader JD, Shugars DA, Makhija S, Vollmer WM: A predictive model for root caries incidence. Caries Res 2016;50:271–278.
35 Sánchez-García S, Reyes-Morales H, Juárez-Cedillo T, Espinel-Bermúdez C, Solórzano-Santos F, García-Peña C: A prediction model for root caries in an elderly population. Community Dent Oral Epidemiol 2011;39:44–52.
36 Sugihara N, Maki Y, Okawa Y, Hosaka M, Matsukubo T, Takaesu Y: Factors associated with root surface caries in elderly. Bull Tokyo Dent Coll 2010;51: 23–30.
37 Ellefsen BS, Morse DE, Waldemar G, Holm-Pedersen P: Indicators for root caries in Danish persons with recently diagnosed Alzheimer's disease. Gerodontology 2012;29:194–202.
38 Islas-Granillo H, Borges-Yañez SA, Medina-Solís CE, Casanova-Rosado AJ, Minaya-Sánchez M, Villalobos Rodelo JJ, Maupomé G: Socioeconomic, sociodemographic, and clinical variables associated with root caries in a group of persons age 60 years and older in Mexico. Geriatr Gerontol Int 2012;12:271–276.
39 Mamai-Homata E, Topitsoglou V, Oulis C, Margaritis V, Polychronopoulou A: Risk indicators of coronal and root caries in Greek middle aged adults and senior citizens. BMC Public Health 2012; 12:484.
40 Gökalp S, Doğan BG: Root caries in 35-44 and 65-74 year-olds in Turkey. Community Dent Health 2012;29:233–238.
41 Ritter AV, Preisser JS, Chung Y, Bader JD, Shugars DA, Amaechi BT, Makhija SK, Funkhouser KA, Vollmer WM; X-ACT Collaborative Research Group: Risk indicators for the presence and extent of root caries among caries-active adults enrolled in the Xylitol for Adult Caries Trial (X-ACT). Clin Oral Investig 2012; 16:1647–1657.
42 Chi DL, Berg JH, Kim AS, Scott J; Northwest Practice-Based REsearch Collaborative in Evidence-based DENTistry: Correlates of root caries experience in middle-aged and older adults in the Northwest Practice-based REsearch Collaborative in Evidence-based DENTistry research network. J Am Dent Assoc 2013;144:507–516.
43 Tan HP, Lo EC: Risk indicators for root caries in institutionalized elders. Community Dent Oral Epidemiol 2014;42: 435–440.
44 Hayes M, Da Mata C, Cole M, McKenna G, Burke F, Allen PF: Risk indicators associated with root caries in independently living older adults. J Dent 2016; 51:8–14.
45 Kumara-Raja B, Radha G: Prevalence of root caries among elders living in residential homes of Bengaluru city, India. J Clin Exp Dent 2016;8:e260–e267.
46 D'Avila OP, Wendland E, Hilgert JB, Padilha DMP, Hugo FN: Association between root caries and depressive symptoms among elders in Carlos Barbosa, RS, Brazil. Braz Dent J 2017;28: 234–240.
47 Hariyani N, Spencer AJ, Luzzi L, Do LG: Root caries experience among Australian adults. Gerodontology 2017; DOI 10.1111/ger.12275.
48 Garton BJ, Ford PJ: Root caries: a survey of Queensland dentists. Int J Dent Hyg 2013;11:216–225.
49 Ismail AI, Pitts NB, Tellez M; Authors of International Caries Classification and Management System (ICCMS™), et al: The International Caries Classification and Management System (ICCMS™) an example of a caries management pathway. BMC Oral Health 2015;15(suppl 1): S9.
50 Pitts N, Ismail AI, Martignon S, Ekstrand K, Douglas GV, Longbottom C: ICCMS™ guide for practitioners and educators. 2014. https://www.icdas.org (accessed June 2017).

Sophie Doméjean
UFR d'Odontologie
2, rue de Braga
FR–63100 Clermont-Ferrand (France)
E-Mail sophie.domejean@uca.fr

Carrilho MRO (ed): Root Caries: From Prevalence to Therapy.
Monogr Oral Sci. Basel, Karger, 2017, vol 26, pp 63–69 (DOI: 10.1159/000479346)

Assessment of Root Caries Lesion Activity and Its Histopathological Features

Thiago Saads Carvalho • Adrian Lussi
Department of Preventive, Restorative and Pediatric Dentistry, University of Bern, Bern, Switzerland

Abstract

Despite certain similarities in the etiology of root caries (RC) and coronal caries, there are notable differences in their histology, namely with regard to the demineralization process, which should be taken into consideration when assessing lesion activity. In this chapter, we present the histological changes to the dentin and pulp, occurring physiologically or in response to caries lesions. We focus on the histological features specific to RC lesions, discussing the assessment of lesion activity. The physiological changes occurring to the dentin and pulp are the formation of secondary dentin and the sclerosis of dentin tubules, while tertiary dentin is formed during pathologic stimuli from caries lesions. Already in the early stages of active RC, the lesions seem softer, and bacteria are easily found within the dentin tubules. Inactive lesions, on the contrary, are characterized by fully remineralized tissue, with irregular mineral precipitation and containing ghost cells of microorganisms. Lesion activity is determined by observing their tactile sensation and their position with respect to the gingival margin.

Introduction

Similarly to coronal caries, root caries (RC) lesions are also characterized according to their activity: as active or inactive (arrested) lesions. However, there are notable differences in the histology of coronal and RC lesions, namely with regard to the demineralization process, and they should be taken into account when assessing their activity. Furthermore, when contemplating the histology of caries lesions, we should also bear in mind the age-related histological changes occurring physiologically to the dentin-pulp complex [1]. In this chapter, we present these histological physiological changes to the dentin and pulp, and we also briefly present some histological changes occurring generally during (coronal and RC) caries lesions. We then describe the histological features specific to RC lesions, focusing on the features specific to active and inactive (arrested) lesions, and finally we discuss the assessment of RC lesion activity.

Histological Changes Occurring Physiologically to the Dentin and Pulp

Carvalho and Lussi [1] described the several changes that occur in both the dentin and the dental pulp with advancing age. A noticeable difference between the dentin from young and elderly individuals is the dentin tubule diameter. Dentin from old teeth (Fig. 1b) are more fibrous, and its

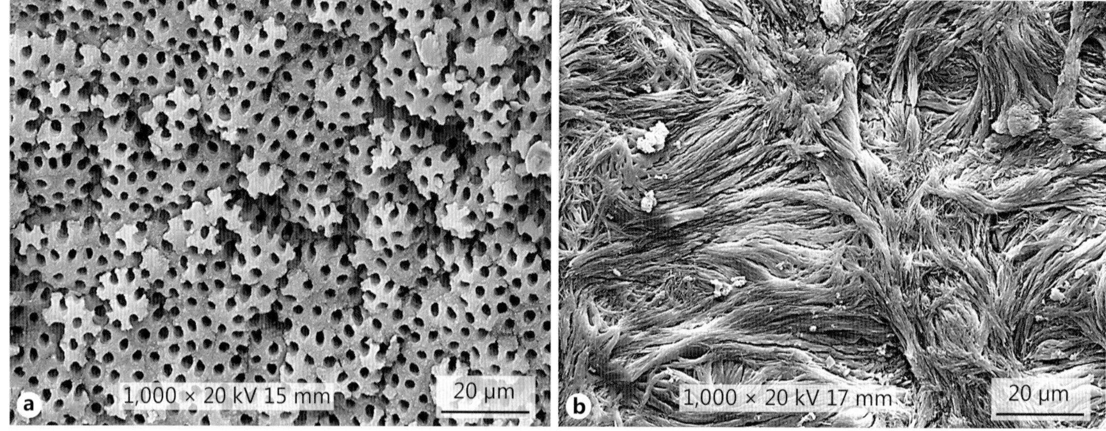

Fig. 1. Scanning electron microscopy images (magnification, ×1,000) of dentin from a young (**a**) and from an older individual (**b**). Open tubules with larger tubular openings in younger dentin (**a**); and fibrous dentin with dentinal tubules almost completely occluded or with very small tubular openings in older dentin (**b**).

tubules are filled with minerals [2], sometimes completely closed up. So dentin from old teeth presents a higher rate of occluded tubules (dentin sclerosis), whereas dentin from young teeth has prominently open tubule lumens (Fig. 1b). In the cervical area, where RC most commonly takes place, Xu et al. [3] reported a significant difference in the tubular area between old and young dentin. Dentin from older individuals (50–80 years old) had significantly smaller tubular area (3.52 ± 0.67 µm) than dentin from younger (17–30 years old) individuals (4.72 ± 0.89 µm) [3].

With the progression of age, secondary dentin is formed. Albeit a slow process, the deposition of secondary dentin on the wall of the pulp chamber is physiological, and begins once the root development is complete and the tooth is fully formed. The deposition of this secondary dentin layer modifies the trajectory of the dentin tubules, and it is also responsible, in parts, for tubule sclerosis.

The formation of secondary dentin also leads to the partial reduction of the volume of the pulp cavity. Therefore, young teeth usually present quite large pulp cavity volumes, but they markedly reduce over the years. A significant reduction in pulp cavity volumes occurs from the age of 22–30 until 51–60 years, but in later age groups (61–70 years), no significant change in volume has been observed [4]. The formation of secondary dentin varies over the years, and it takes place primarily on the distal and mesial walls of the pulp cavity, leading to a reduction in the volume of the pulp in the mesial-distal direction [5, 6] mirrored in x-rays. In older age groups, the volume of the pulp cavity also decreases in the vestibular-oral direction, due to the formation of fibrous dentin [5]. Additionally, a small, but significant difference in pulp cavity volume has been reported between genders [7].

The formation of secondary dentin, as well as tubule sclerosis, lead to a considerable decrease in fluid movement within the dentin tubules [8], which, in turn, leads to a decrease in pulp sensibility in older individuals.

Histological Changes Generally Occurring during Caries Lesions

Caries lesions are pathologic stimuli that incite the production of tertiary dentin. Tertiary dentin is characterized as either reactionary or reparative

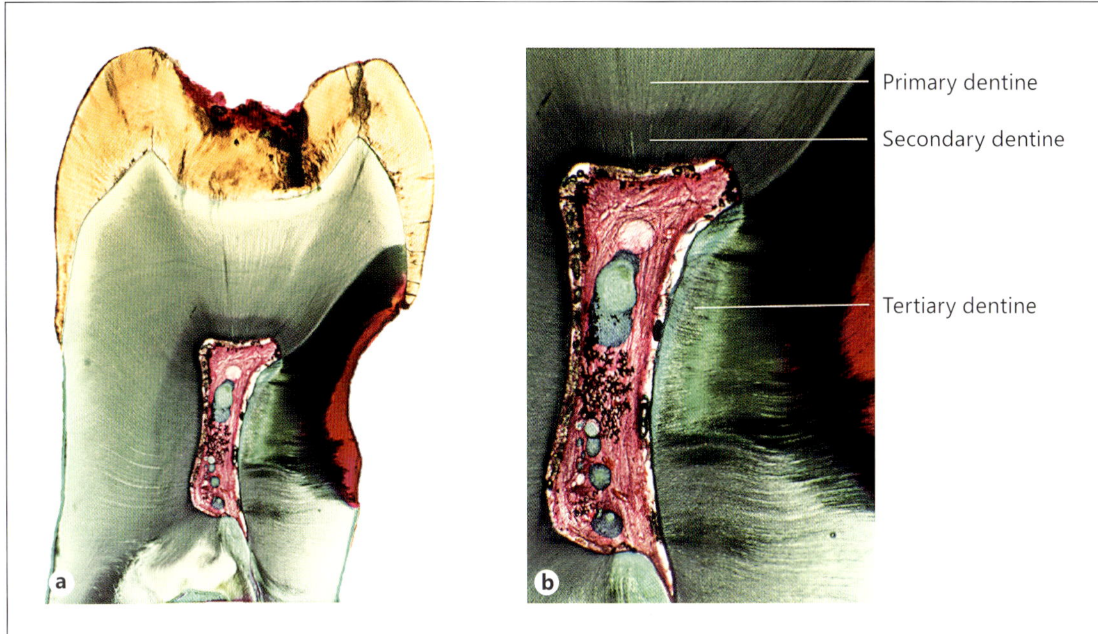

Fig. 2. Histological cross-section of molar presenting a root caries lesion extending into dentin (**a**). Magnification of the lesion (**b**), highlighting the details of primary, secondary, and tertiary dentin. The latter is differentiated into reactionary tertiary dentin (containing tubules), and reparative tertiary dentin (atubular and directly adjacent to the pulp cavity). Note the presence of dental pulp stones (dental pulp calculi) in the pulp tissue, a typical occurrence in older patients.

dentin, depending on the stimuli type. Reactionary dentin is formed in response to milder stimuli. Such stimuli activate primary odontoblasts that already exist in the dentino-pulp complex into depositing new dentin tissue onto the pulpal wall. Reactionary dentin also presents traces of dentin tubules because it is produced by odontoblasts. Conversely, reparative dentin is produced in response to more severe pathologic stimuli. Such stimuli destroy the primary odontoblast layer and trigger mesenchymal cells in the pulp to migrate to the dentin wall and rapidly produce reparative dentin. Due to its accelerated deposition, reparative dentin is atubular (has no dentin tubules), may exhibit a bone-like structure (osteodentin), and may present traces of cells in its matrix [1]. Tertiary dentin in RC lesions can be observed in Figures 2 and 3.

Histological Features Specific to RC Lesions

Features Specific to Active RC Lesions

Despite certain similarities in the etiology of active RC and coronal caries, their histopathology is rather different. A major distinction is that the root surface is covered by a very thin layer of cementum and, during the RC process, bacteria can already be found within the dentin tubules at the initial stages of the caries development [9, 10]. Moreover, RC lesions seem softer at an earlier stage in the caries process in comparison to coronal caries [11].

For RC lesions to develop, some degree of gingival recession is required, and the caries lesions themselves occur mainly on a supragingival region [12]. As cariogenic plaque accumulates on the root surface, initial demineralization of the cementum takes place.

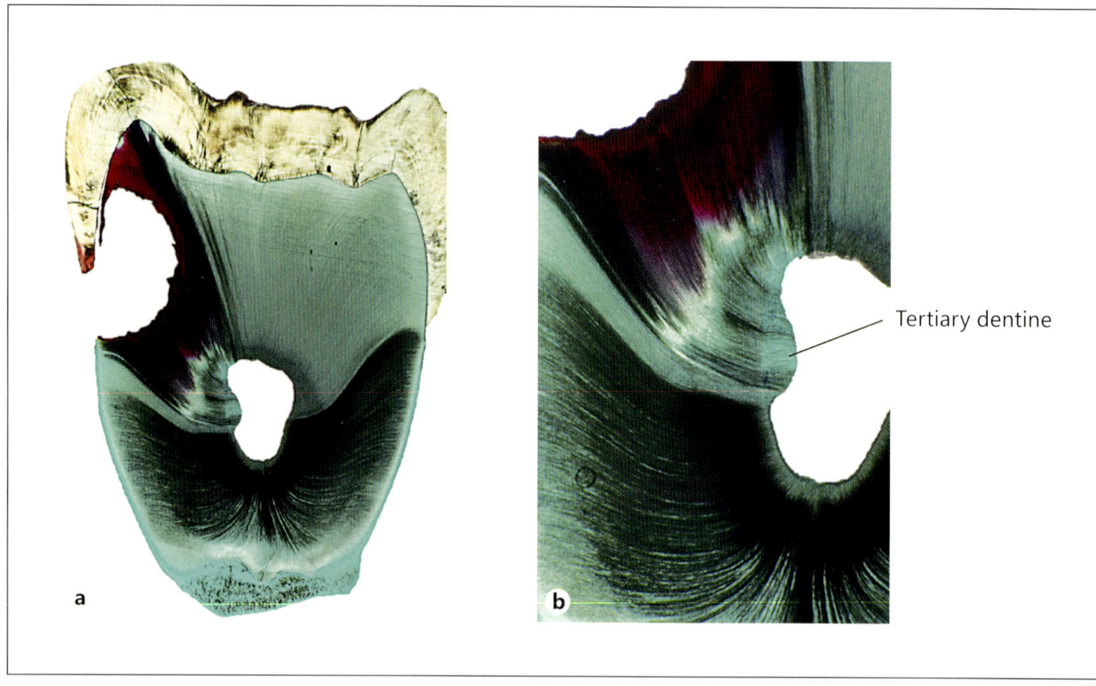

Fig. 3. Histological cross-section of molar presenting a root caries lesion extending into dentin (**a**) and magnification of the lesion (**b**).

It has been reported that the thickness of cementum continuously increases with age [13]. However, this expansion occurs at much slower rates in cervical areas of the tooth, where the cementum layer is the narrowest, varying from 54 µm (at ages between 11 and 20 years) to 128 µm (between 51 and 76 years) [13], which explains the fact that the caries lesions invade the underlying dentin at much earlier stages than in coronal caries. Moreover, in cases of periodontal patients, or those presenting calculus, the continuous root scaling throughout lifetime can considerably reduce the thickness of the cementum, possibly exposing the underlying dentin and leaving the root surface more susceptible.

During the early stages of RC lesion formation, if cementum is still present, small clefts appear along this tissue [14], which becomes filled with microorganisms. These clefts can cut across the whole cementum layer and reach the subjacent dentin tissue. The penetration of microorganisms into the cementum and, eventually, into the dentin occurs mostly along these clefts [15].

As the microorganisms penetrate deeper into the cementum, the demineralization induces a broadening of clefts [14], thus weakening the cementum structure, and ultimately leading to microscopic fissures that expose the underlying dentin. However, part of the cementum surface remains mineralized, so the initial RC lesions are also characterized by a subsurface demineralization, observed as a radiolucent area in radiographs [12]. At this stage, Schupbach et al. [15] reported that the demineralization occurs most frequently in a uniform pattern.

As the early lesion breaks through the cementum, the demineralization front reaches the underlying dentin tissue. This immediate subjacent dentin (approximately 150 µm below the cemento-dentin junction) is made up mostly of sclerotic/atubular dentin [14]. The initial demineralization causes a loss of minerals of the atubular dentin, but leaves most of the organic matrix (collagen) intact. This collagen layer will remain part of the lesion until it is either degraded by host-derived proteolytic enzymes, such as collagenase or other proteinases, or removed mechanically [12]. As the lesion progresses further into the dentin, we observe greater loss of the cementum, and eventually a loss of the surface contour [12], leaving the dentin exposed to the oral cavity. At this stage, small clefts are also observed in the atubular dentin. These clefts also serve as passageways for microorganisms to penetrate even further into the atubular dentin [15], and ultimately reach the dentin tubules, located deeper in the tissue.

The expansion of the demineralization front causes a further increase in the size of the caries lesion, exposing a greater area of the dentin to the oral cavity, and upholding the progression of the lesion into more advanced stages. In such more advanced caries lesions, the microorganisms reach the tubules, and are able to invade even deeper into the dentin [16], causing a destruction of the inner part of the peritubular dentin and demineralization of the intertubular dentin [15]. It has been suggested that this process could also be driven forward by the dentinal fluid, which may act as a source of proteolytic enzymes [17]. The demineralization of the intertubular dentin provides leeway for microorganisms to spread laterally between the dentin tubules, promoting additional mineral loss and further damage to the organic matrix, thus characterizing a "soft" active lesion [18]. Therefore, at this stage, the active lesion is deeper than 150 μm and it clearly presents a soft sensation to probing.

It is noteworthy that, on the deep end of the dentin lesions, closer to the dental pulp, a mineralized area can be observed. In this area, Wefel et al. [19] detected that the course of the dentin tubules is disrupted and the tubules themselves are less prominent. Schupbach et al. [15] explained that this mineralized band in the periphery of the dentinal caries lesion is the outcome of tubule sclerosis, where the intertubular dentin is partially mineralized with large crystals similar to hydroxyapatite. So, sclerosis of dentin tubules also occurs as a response to cariogenic stimuli in RC.

Features Specific to Inactive (Arrested) RC Lesions

Since RC is a process driven forward by the cariogenic biofilm, a shift in the biofilm equilibrium through regular toothbrushing and use of fluoride-containing toothpastes can delay or even inactivate (arrest) the carious process [11]. This has been clinically demonstrated by Nyvad and Fejerskov [20], who showed that, after 2–3 months of daily toothbrushing with fluoride toothpaste, RC lesions presented initial signs of arrest. Also, Souza et al. [21] suggested that RC lesions have greater chances of inactivation when the patients present fewer RC lesions, and when the lesions themselves have less plaque, smaller surface area, and are farther away from the gingival margin [21].

It is important to bear in mind that caries is a dynamic demineralization and remineralization process. In this regard, Schupbach et al. [15] remarked that, within the same lesion, it is possible to observe areas of active caries, areas of inactive caries, as well as areas of remineralization, thus illustrating the difficulty in distinguishing between lesions in the initial stages of inactivation (remineralizing) and lesions that still sustain active demineralization. However, once the lesions are actually inactive, they present some specific histologic aspects.

The main characteristic of inactive lesions is the presence of a distinctly mineralized, hard surface layer. Also, the lesion is separated from the underlying sound dentin by a distinct layer of sclerotic dentin [22]. Schupbach et al. [15] advocate that this sclerotic layer is an advanced guard between the demineralization front and the dental pulp, and it is a fundamental condition for successful lesion inactivation.

Table 1. Diagnostic criteria for assessing root caries lesion activity (based on [23])

	Tactile sensation	Position of the lesion
Active lesions	Soft or leathery on probing	Close to the gingival margin
Inactive (arrested) lesions	Hard on probing	Distant from the gingival margin

Another typical aspect of inactivated lesions is that the dentin tubules present intratubular mineralization with an irregular precipitation pattern [15], and ghost cells of microorganisms are present between these crystals. Concomitantly, the intertubular dentin also presents itself fully remineralized up to the surface of the lesion [22]. Furthermore, as previously mentioned, a zone of dentin sclerosis is clearly identified in the interface between the inactive lesion and the underlying sound dentin [22].

Assessment of RC Lesion Activity

The assessment of the activity of RC lesions has been classically done according to their visual appearance (color) and tactile sensation. Based on color, RC lesions with a yellowish to brown appearance were generally classified as active, whereas lesions with a brownish to black appearance were typically classified as inactive. However, Lynch and Beighton [18] associated the tactile sensation of RC lesions with respect to their color and distance from the gingival margin. Remarkably, the authors found that color is not a useful diagnosis criterion for activity, but rather distance from the gingival margin is a useful criterion. The authors observed that active (soft) lesions developed closest to the gingival margin, whereas inactive (hard) lesions were found farthest away from the gingiva [18].

Nyvad et al. [23] propose a diagnostic criteria (Table 1), based mainly on tactile sensation and the position from the gingival margin. Active lesions are soft or leathery, and are found at plaque retention sites close to the gingival margin or along the cemento-enamel junction; inactive (arrested) lesions are hard on probing, present a shiny appearance, and lie within some distance from the gingival margin [23].

While assessing lesion activity, it is important to bear in mind that, within the same lesion, it is possible to find active and inactive areas, as well as areas undergoing remineralization. Therefore, during an examination of a clinically sound root surface, it may be possible to observe areas of unaltered tissue interspersed with areas of demineralization [9]. Crucially, dental professionals should also look for other causative factors related to the caries disease, such as the presence of plaque, cariogenic diet, gingival bleeding, among many others. A timely and correct assessment of RC lesions will promote the best chances for the patients, preventing new lesions from forming or preventing existing lesions from progressing [24].

Conclusion

Despite a similar etiology between coronal caries and RC, the latter presents distinct peculiarities concerning its histology. Fully understanding the histology of RC lesion progression may allow for a better comprehension of the cariogenic process and lesion activity. The assessment of lesion activity should be mainly based on tactile sensation and position of the lesion with respect to the gingival margin. In short, active lesions are soft/leathery, and found close to the gingival margin; inactive lesions are hard, and lie within some distance from the gingival margin.

Disclosure Statement

No ethical approval was necessary for the present manuscript. This study was self-funded by the Department of Preventive, Restorative and Pediatric Dentistry. The authors declare no conflict of interest.

Acknowledgements

The authors wish to thank Brigitte Megert, Isabel Hug, and Dr. Hermann Stich for their efforts in obtaining the figures used in this chapter.

References

1 Carvalho TS, Lussi A: Age-related morphological, histological and functional changes in teeth. J Oral Rehabil 2017;44:291–298.
2 Ryou H, Romberg E, Pashley DH, Tay FR, Arola D: Importance of age on the dynamic mechanical behavior of intertubular and peritubular dentin. J Mech Behav Biomed Mater 2015;42:229–242.
3 Xu H, Zheng Q, Shao Y, et al: The effects of ageing on the biomechanical properties of root dentine and fracture. J Dent 2014;42:305–311.
4 Porto LV, Celestino da Silva Neto J, Anjos Pontual AD, Catunda RQ: Evaluation of volumetric changes of teeth in a Brazilian population by using cone beam computed tomography. J Forensic Leg Med 2015;36:4–9.
5 Schroeder HE: [Age-related changes in the pulp chamber and its wall in human canine teeth]. Schweiz Monatsschr Zahnmed 1993;103:141–149.
6 Schroeder HE, Krey G, Preisig E: [Age-related changes of the pulpal dentin wall in human front teeth]. Schweiz Monatsschr Zahnmed 1990;100:1450–1461.
7 Ge ZP, Yang P, Li G, Zhang JZ, Ma XC: Age estimation based on pulp cavity/chamber volume of 13 types of tooth from cone beam computed tomography images. Int J Legal Med 2016;130:1159–1167.
8 Thaler A, Ebert J, Petschelt A, Pelka M: Influence of tooth age and root section on root dentine dye penetration. Int Endod J 2008;41:1115–1122.
9 Nyvad B, Fejerskov O: Root surface caries: clinical, histopathological and microbiological features and clinical implications. Int Dent J 1982;32:311–326.
10 Ekstrand KR, Zero DT, Martignon S, Pitts NB: Lesion activity assessment. Monogr Oral Sci 2009;21:63–90.
11 Kidd EA, Fejerskov O: What constitutes dental caries? Histopathology of carious enamel and dentin related to the action of cariogenic biofilms. J Dent Res 2004;83:C35–C38.
12 Wefel JS: Root caries histopathology and chemistry. Am J Dent 1994;7:261–265.
13 Zander HA, Hurzeler B: Continuous cementum apposition. J Dent Res 1958;37:1035–1044.
14 Schüpbach P, Guggenheim B, Lutz F: Human root caries: histopathology of initial lesions in cementum and dentin. J Oral Pathol Med 1989;18:146–156.
15 Schüpbach P, Guggenheim B, Lutz F: Histopathology of root surface caries. J Dent Res 1990;69:1195–1204.
16 Schüpbach P, Guggenheim B, Lutz F: Human root caries: histopathology of advanced lesions. Caries Res 1990;24:145–158.
17 Tjäderhane L, Buzalaf MA, Carrilho M, Chaussain C: Matrix metalloproteinases and other matrix proteinases in relation to cariology: the era of 'dentin degradomics'. Caries Res 2015;49:193–208.
18 Lynch E, Beighton D: A comparison of primary root caries lesions classified according to colour. Caries Res 1994;28:233–239.
19 Wefel JS, Clarkson BH, Heilman JR: Natural root caries: a histologic and microradiographic evaluation. J Oral Pathol 1985;14:615–623.
20 Nyvad B, Fejerskov O: Active root surface caries converted into inactive caries as a response to oral hygiene. Scand J Dent Res 1986;94:281–284.
21 Souza ML, Cury JA, Tenuta LM, et al: Comparing the efficacy of a dentifrice containing 1.5% arginine and 1450 ppm fluoride to a dentifrice containing 1450 ppm fluoride alone in the management of primary root caries. J Dent 2013;41(suppl 2):S35–S41.
22 Schüpbach P, Lutz F, Guggenheim B: Human root caries: histopathology of arrested lesions. Caries Res 1992;26:153–164.
23 Nyvad B, Machiulskiene V, Soviero VM, Baelum V: Visual-tactile caries diagnosis; in Fejerskov O, Nyvad B, Kidd E (eds): Dental Caries: The Disease and Its Clinical Management, ed 3. Chichester, UK, John Wiley & Sons, 2015, pp 191–209.
24 Rodrigues JA, Lussi A, Seemann R, Neuhaus KW: Prevention of crown and root caries in adults. Periodontol 2000 2011;55:231–249.

Thiago Saads Carvalho
Department of Preventive, Restorative and Pediatric Dentistry, University of Bern
Freiburgstrasse 7
CH–3010 Bern (Switzerland)
E-Mail thiago.saads@zmk.unibe.ch

Carrilho MRO (ed): Root Caries: From Prevalence to Therapy.
Monogr Oral Sci. Basel, Karger, 2017, vol 26, pp 70–75 (DOI: 10.1159/000479347)

Monitoring of Root Caries Lesions

Iain A. Pretty

Division of Dentistry, Faculty of Biology, Medicine and Health, The University of Manchester, Manchester, UK

Abstract

The early detection of root caries is essential for the implementation of appropriate preventive therapeutic regimes. Subsequent monitoring of lesions is required to determine the outcomes of such therapies. While much research activity has been seen in the detection and monitoring of enamel caries, this has not been seen in root caries – despite the possibilities for shorter clinical trials due to the more rapid remineralization and arrest of such lesions. The main stay of both clinical practice and research has been the use of visual tactile criteria including, hardness, texture, the presence or absence of cavitation, and color. A range of clinical trials, using high fluoride products of known efficacy, have shown such techniques to be valid. The use of adjunct technologies has been limited in large scale in vivo studies, to devices using electrical resistance measurement (electronic caries monitor, ECM). The use of dyes, laser fluorescence, and advanced imaging such as near infra-red has been described in vitro but few, with the exception of DiagnoDent, have been translated to chair side. Except for ECM, no other technology has been used in the clinical assessments of root caries remineralization and there remains a need to supplement visual tactile techniques for future work.

Introduction

Once detected, and appropriate therapies introduced, there is a need to monitor root caries lesions to determine the efficacy of treatment in both clinical practice and clinical trials. In enamel caries, there is a wealth of research describing a range of visual, tactile, and technological-based methods for lesion progression, arrest, and reversal. When considering root caries, there is a relatively smaller number of techniques available, especially for use in general clinical practice, and visual tactile methods remain the predominant means of monitoring such lesions. Dental radiographs have little value in detecting root caries lesions at an early stage. The following chapter describes the existing and emerging methods for the assessment of root caries lesions.

Visual Tactile Methods

The assessment of root lesions by visual and/or tactile measurement remains the commonest means for both detecting and monitoring root caries lesions [1]. There are a range of physical phenomenon that can be assessed including texture, location, the presence and absence of cavitation, surface contour, and the reflectance of light [2]. The use of color to determine the activity of root caries lesions, once thought to be highly predictive, has now largely been disregarded [3] although authorities still recognize its value in the detection of caries [4], and it continues to feature in root caries indices. The scientific basis for the use of each of these elements has been extensively described by Lynch and coworkers in a series of papers, looking at microbiological validation [5], the use of color [4], treatment need [6], and both mechanical and electrical factors [7].

The early detection of root caries can be more complex compared to enamel caries as the early white spot lesion, seen on air drying, is not present. Banting [8] argues that the presence or absence of cavitation (or loss of surface continuity) is not a prerequisite for the diagnosis of root caries but that the detection of "softening" has wide acceptance as a criteria of caries. The location of the suspected lesion is also important with active root caries lesions occurring at plaque retention sites close to the gingival margin. Proximity to the gingival margin is the result of attachment loss and exposure of dentin leading to an increased caries risk. The reflectance of lesions is an important diagnostic criterion for activity – with matt lesions being more frequently associated with an active caries process and shiny lesions being associated with arrest [9].

The formalization of visual and tactile criteria into caries classification systems such as ICDAS has been slow, with proposed criteria but little validation [10]. Much of the published literature on root caries assessment has been concerned with the detection of lesions, rather than the monitoring of their natural history over time. This lack of research reflects the difficulty in undertaking clinical research on older adults [11]. An exception to this is the work of Baysan et al. [12] and Ekstrand et al. [13, 14].

Table 1. Ekstrand's scoring system for root caries activity – brackets indicate the value to be allocated to each finding after [14]

Criterion	Finding
Texture of the lesion when gently probed	
	Hard (0)
	Leathery (2)
	Soft (3)
Contour of the surface	
	No cavitation or the surroundings of the cavity smooth to probing (1)
	Cavitation with irregular boarder (2)
Distance from the lesion to the gingival margin	
	‡1 mm from the gingiva margin (1)
	<1 mm from the gingiva margin (2)
Color of the lesion	
	Dark brown/black (1)
	Light brown/yellowish (2)

In his 2001 study, Baysan et al. [12] used a combination of hardness, cavitation, size, color, and plaque coverage to assess remineralization of lesions following the application of dentifrices of differing fluoride concentration (5,000 and 1,100 ppm) [12]. An assessment of lesions was also undertaken using electrical impedance, which is discussed later in this chapter. Baysan et al. [12] found that there was a two-fold increase in lesions becoming hardened in the high fluoride group compared to the control and that the cavitation status of the lesion at baseline was an important predictor of the ability to remineralize and arrest lesions.

Ekstrand et al. [14] developed a scoring system to determine the activity of root caries lesions in a clinical trial assessing different therapeutic regimes. The scoring system is shown in Table 1.

The scores for each lesion are calculated, and a score of 3–5 is considered as an arrested lesion and 6–9 as active. The thresholds were assessed for both accuracy and reproducibility, and the scoring system was used in a subsequent clinical trial of a high fluoride toothpaste (5,000 ppm) compared to a standard (1,450 ppm) paste [13]. Using the scoring system to describe the activity, it was shown that the high fluoride group had significantly more arrested lesions than the regular fluoride group, demonstrating construct validity for the scoring system.

A simpler approach was taken in another study examining the use of high fluorides in the management of root caries [15]. In this study, the assessment of lesions was limited to surface hardness using the following scale:

Level 1: Hard
Level 2: Hard to leathery
Level 3: Leathery
Level 4: Leathery with local softening
Level 5: Soft

The authors reported significant differences in hardness scores between the control paste (1,350 ppm) and the higher fluoride group at 3 and 6 months. The use of a high fluoride intervention in the study lends biological plausibility to the use of hardness as a measure of remineralization and arrest.

Challenges

There is evidence that various visual and tactile criteria can be used to both detect and then subsequently monitor root caries lesions. However, like all visual tactile methods they are subjective, and while they may be simple to deploy in detecting lesions, their use for longitudinal monitoring is more complex as there is a requirement to record changes. For example, while it may be a simple matter to describe a lesion as "soft" on a clinical assessment – how can a clinician record a difference in "softness" at a subsequent visit? Visual tactile methods do not permit the discrimination of lesions with or without a remineralized surface layer [16].

These challenges have also been identified in enamel caries monitoring that has led to the development of numerous technologies to not only detect lesions earlier, but also to monitor their status over time. Like enamel caries, early detection of root lesions is essential if prevention is to be effective (note the impact of cavitation on the prediction of arrest in Ekstrand's work [13]) and measurement of the effect of therapies is important in both clinical practice and trials of new products. The development of technologies to detect and monitor progression of root caries has not mirrored the exponential interest in enamel caries technologies. As such there are limited options for clinicians or researchers who wish to adopt more objective measures into their work.

Electronic Caries Monitor

Electronic caries monitoring is based on the measurement of electrical resistance of the tooth structure during controlled drying. Electrical resistance increases as the pore volume of dentin decreases – and hence, the remineralization of dentin can be related to electronic caries monitor (ECM) measurements [17]. ECM has been used in clinical trials of root caries remineralization where after 3 and 6 months use of a high fluoride toothpaste, significant differences were seen in ECM resistance values [12]. The ECM device has been the most frequently used root caries monitoring technology within clinical trials, although it has little application in clinical practice. The system is operator-sensitive and, as a point measurement, requires the careful repositioning of the monitor tip in the same recording position to ensure reliability over longitudinal measurements [18]. In clinical trials, there are generally 5 measurements for each lesion, using a North, South, East, West, and Centre approach [17] (Fig. 1, 2).

While the current implementation of ECM restricts its use to clinical trials, the underlying principle of resistance measurement is well validated in vivo [19] and hence could form the basis for future practice-based assessment device [20].

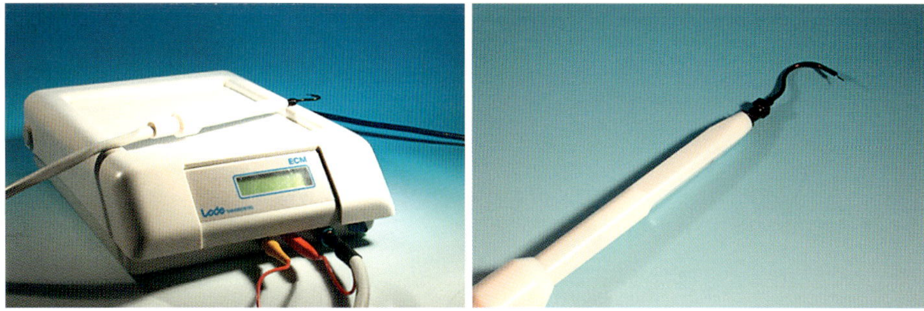

Fig. 1. The electronic caries monitor equipment.

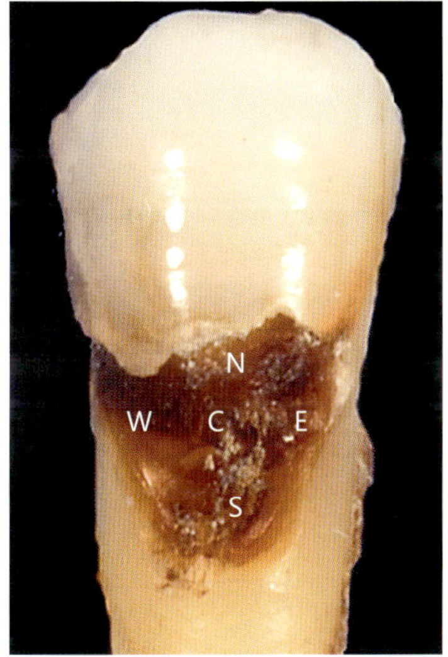

Fig. 2. Example of sampling a lesion by electronic caries monitor point measurement using north (N), south (S), east (E), west (W), and centre measurement points, within the lesion.

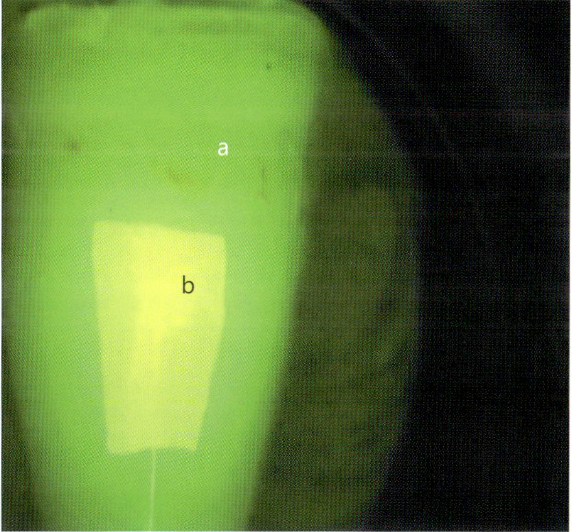

Fig. 3. Example of an artificial root lesion with fluorescein dye under QLF conditions. Area (a) represents sound, no demineralized enamel, whereas area (b) shows the artificial lesion with higher levels of fluorescence due to dye penetration.

Dye-Enhanced Methods

The increased porosity seen in active root caries lesions [8] offers an opportunity to use dyes to measure the degree and extent of porosity. The use of fluorescein has been described, initially by van der Veen and ten Bosch [16] – who reported a good correlation between dye penetration and the lesion's mineral status in both natural and artificial lesions [21]. Pretty combined this work with the use of quantitative light-induced fluorescence to provide a means of quantifying the uptake of fluorescein and found similar levels of correlation with mineral loss [22] (Fig. 3).

Despite the safety profile of fluorescein and its use in other medical applications, this initial work has not extended into the in vivo application of dye-enhanced root caries monitoring.

DiagnoDent

While the use of the DiagnoDent (DD) device for enamel caries has little supporting evidence [23, 24], the device has been proposed as a useful tool for the assessment of root caries [25]. DD measurements in enamel caries are often confounded by the presence of stain and the complex morphology of the fissure system on occlusal lesions [19]. The simpler root surface may, therefore, negate some of these confounding factors. In vitro work with natural root surface lesions found moderate correlation between DD scores and histological depth. Like enamel, the DD readings were confounded by stain, where black, shallow lesions resulted in higher DD values [19].

An in vivo study by Zhang et al. [26] examined root caries on 266 subjects using DD and visual tactile methods. This initial study provides promising results with significant differences reported in DD values for sound and carious root surfaces. For those surfaces categorized as carious, there were also significant differences between active and inactive lesions. The authors recognized that the work was preliminary and that the biological explanations for the differences in laser fluorescence values as well as further histological validation would need to be undertaken [26].

Other Methods

There have been a number of other methods suggested for root caries monitoring that are either in their infancy or rarely used. Ekstrand used Clin-Pro (3M ESPE) impression materials to detect lactic acid production by root caries lesions [14] as a means of validation in his clinical study. A recent search found that the impression material is no longer marketed.

A very recent study described the use of near infrared, thermal imaging, and optical coherence tomography for root lesion activity assessment using both bovine and natural root lesions [27], and compared it to a clinical assessment using ICDAS II. The optical coherence tomography method and the thermal imaging approaches both demonstrated utility although the near infrared was adversely affected by the anatomy of lesions and their severity.

Conclusion

The combination of hardness, location, cavitation, and shine as indicators of both the presence and status of root caries lesions remains the predominant means of detecting and monitoring root caries lesions in clinical practice. The problems of recording such features within clinical records complicates the process of longitudinal monitoring of such lesions, although the use of intra-oral white light photography may enable some assessment of lesion progression [28]. The subjective nature of these measurements, while recognized, is moderated by the relatively rapid de- and remineralization processes of root caries and the combination of factors demonstrating an arrested lesion – that is, the presence of hardened, shiny dentin. In addition, there are a multitude of studies that have employed visual and tactile criteria successfully, lending significant construct validity to the measures – especially those using hardness as an outcome measure.

Within clinical trials of root caries lesions, ECM remains the predominant technology-based methodology, and the link between lesion porosity and the surface's electrical resistance offers a potential for future device measurement. Developments in optical- and laser-based systems offer future potential, but require further research before they can be adopted into mainstream practice. Research on patients with root surface lesions is complicated – not least as the epidemiology suggests that those patients at highest risk are nursing and care home residents. Such trials are expensive and commercially there is little imperative to undertake them. However, if diagnostic tests are to be developed and assessed, then such barriers must be overcome. For now, the use of carefully applied visual and tactile assessment, combined with, if necessary, ECM, are the most evidenced means of assessing root caries progression and arrest.

References

1 Katz RV: Clinical signs of root caries: measurement issues. J Dent Res 1990; 69:1211–1215.
2 Fejerskov O, Luan WM, Nyvad B, Budtz-Jørgensen E, Holm-Pedersen P: Active and inactive root surface caries lesions in a selected group of 60- to 80-year-old Danes. Caries Res 1991;25:385–391.
3 Hellyer PH, Beighton D, Heath MR, Lynch EJ: Root caries in older people attending a general dental practice in East Sussex. Br Dent J 1990;169:201–206.
4 Lynch E, Beighton D: A comparison of primary root caries lesions classified according to colour. Caries Res 1994;28: 233–239.
5 Beighton D, Lynch E: Comparison of selected microflora of plaque and underlying carious dentine associated with primary root caries lesions. Caries Res 1995;29:154–158.
6 Beighton D, Lynch E, Heath MR: A microbiological study of primary root-caries lesions with different treatment needs. J Dent Res 1993;72:623–629.
7 Baysan A, Prinz JF, Lynch E: Clinical criteria used to detect primary root caries with electrical and mechanical measurements in vitro. Am J Dent 2004;17:94–98.
8 Banting DW: The diagnosis of root caries. J Dent Educ 2001;65:991–996.
9 Rodrigues JA, Lussi A, Seemann R, Neuhaus KW: Prevention of crown and root caries in adults. Periodontol 2000 2011; 55:231–249.
10 Ismail AI, Sohn W, Tellez M, Amaya A, Sen A, Hasson H, et al: The International Caries Detection and Assessment System (ICDAS): an integrated system for measuring dental caries. Community Dent Oral Epidemiol 2007;35:170–178.
11 Pretty IA, Ellwood RP, Lo EC, MacEntee MI, Müller F, Rooney E, et al: The Seattle Care Pathway for securing oral health in older patients. Gerodontology 2014;31(suppl 1):77–87.
12 Baysan A, Lynch E, Ellwood R, Davies R, et al: Reversal of primary root caries using dentifrices containing 5,000 and 1,100 ppm fluoride. Caries Res 2001;35:41–46.
13 Ekstrand KR, Poulsen JE, Hede B, Twetman S, Qvist V, Ellwood RP: A Randomized clinical trial of the anti-caries efficacy of 5,000 compared to 1,450 ppm fluoridated toothpaste on root caries lesions in elderly disabled nursing home residents. Caries Res 2013;47:391–398.
14 Ekstrand K, Martignon S, Holm-Pedersen P: Development and evaluation of two root caries controlling programmes for home-based frail people older than 75 years. Gerodontology 2008;25:67–75.
15 Srinivasan M, Schimmel M, Riesen M, Ilgner A, Wicht MJ, Warncke M, et al: High-fluoride toothpaste: a multicenter randomized controlled trial in adults. Community Dent Oral Epidemiol 2014; 42:333–340.
16 van der Veen MH, ten Bosch JJ: An in vitro evaluation of fluorescein penetration into natural root surface carious lesions. Caries Res 1993;27:258–261.
17 Petersson LG, Kambara M: Remineralisation study of artificial root caries lesions after fluoride treatment. An in vitro study using electric caries monitor and transversal micro-radiography. Gerodontology 2004;21:85–92.
18 Petersson LG, Magnusson K, Hakestam U, Baigi A, Twetman S: Reversal of primary root caries lesions after daily intake of milk supplemented with fluoride and probiotic lactobacilli in older adults. Acta Odontol Scand 2011;69:321–327.
19 Wicht MJ, Haak R, Stützer H, Strohe D, Noack MJ: Intra- and interexaminer variability and validity of laser fluorescence and electrical resistance readings on root surface lesions. Caries Res 2002; 36:241–248.
20 Pretty IA, Ellwood RP: The caries continuum: opportunities to detect, treat and monitor the re-mineralization of early caries lesions. J Dent 2013;41(suppl 2):S12–S21.
21 van der Veen MH, Tsuda H, Arends J, ten Bosch JJ: Evaluation of sodium fluorescein for quantitative diagnosis of root caries. J Dent Res 1996;75:588–593.
22 Pretty IA, Ingram GS, Agalamanyi EA, Edgar WM, Higham SM: The use of fluorescein-enhanced quantitative light-induced fluorescence to monitor de- and re-mineralization of in vitro root caries. J Oral Rehabil 2003;30:1151–1156.
23 Gomez J, Tellez M, Pretty IA, Ellwood RP, Ismail AI: Non-cavitated carious lesions detection methods: a systematic review. Community Dent Oral Epidemiol 2013;41:54–66.
24 Bader JD, Shugars DA: A systematic review of the performance of a laser fluorescence device for detecting caries. J Am Dent Assoc 2004;135:1413–1426.
25 Haak R, Wicht MJ: Caries detection and quantification with DIAGNOdent: prospects for occlusal and root caries? Int J Comput Dent 2004;7:347–358.
26 Zhang W, McGrath C, Lo EC: A comparison of root caries diagnosis based on visual-tactile criteria and DIAGNOdent in vivo. J Dent 2009;37:509–513.
27 Lee RC, Darling CL, Staninec M, Ragadio A, Fried D: Activity assessment of root caries lesions with thermal and near-IR imaging methods. J Biophotonics 2017;10:433–445.
28 Birch S, Bridgman C, Brocklehurst P, Ellwood R, Gomez J, Helgeson M, et al: Prevention in practice – a summary. BMC Oral Health 2015;15(suppl 1):S12.

Prof. Iain A. Pretty
The University of Manchester, Dental Health Unit
Williams House, Manchester Science Park
Manchester M16 6SE (UK)
E-Mail iain.pretty@manchester.ac.uk

Carrilho MRO (ed): Root Caries: From Prevalence to Therapy.
Monogr Oral Sci. Basel, Karger, 2017, vol 26, pp 76–82 (DOI: 10.1159/000479348)

Biofilm Control and Oral Hygiene Practices

Marisa Maltz[a] • Luana Severo Alves[b] • Julio Eduardo do Amaral Zenkner[b]

[a]Federal University of Rio Grande do Sul, Porto Alegre, and [b]Federal University of Santa Maria, Santa Maria, Brazil

Abstract

As the thick biofilm in the presence of fermentable carbohydrates is the main etiological factor of dental caries, the frequent and systematic removal of this colony by means of an effective biofilm control should result in the prevention of caries lesions or in the arrest of the local carious process. However, the role of biofilm control in the management of dental caries has been questioned. This chapter will discuss the biofilm control and oral hygiene practices on root surfaces. Laboratory and clinical studies describing the effect of biofilm control and oral hygiene practices on the arrestment of root carious lesions are described. Epidemiological surveys evaluating the association between oral hygiene and root caries are discussed. Finally, some aspects on chemical biofilm control are also presented.

Introduction

Dental caries is a multifactorial disease whose main biologic determinant is the dental biofilm. It causes a chemical dissolution of dental tissues due to the presence of acids that are derived from the fermentation of sugar by microorganism of the dental biofilm. On the contrary, while dental biofilm is essential for the development and progression of dental caries, it is not sufficient for the disease to occur. As the thick biofilm in the presence of fermentable carbohydrates is a key etiological factor for dental caries, the frequent and systematic removal of this colony of microorganisms by means of an effective biofilm control should result in the prevention or in the arrestment of caries lesions. However, the role of biofilm control (mechanical and chemical) in the management of dental caries has been questioned since conflicting results have been reported.

This chapter will discuss the biofilm control and oral hygiene practices on root surfaces. It is important to recognize that the formation of a root carious lesion differs, in some important aspects, from the development of coronal caries, as described in the chapter by Damé-Teixeira et al., this volume, pp. 15–25. Enamel carious lesions progress reflecting the direction of enamel prisms, and due to its high mineral content, usually present sharp limits at the surface angle. In general, the depth of coronal lesions tends to exceed its width, thus resulting in a retentive cavity commonly inaccessible for cleaning by the patient. Conversely, root lesions, mainly located in dentin, progress shallowly, usually resulting in saucer-shaped cavities. The expulsive configuration of root lesions simplifies the mechanical removal and control of dental biofilm. Usually, such lesions are easily accessible to the patient.

Laboratory and clinical studies describing the effect of biofilm control and oral hygiene practices on the arrestment of root carious lesions are described in this chapter. Epidemiological surveys evaluating the association between oral hygiene and root caries are discussed. Finally, some aspects of chemical biofilm control are also presented.

It is important to point out that the introduction of fluoridated dentifrices in the second half of 20th century has somehow disturbed the possibility of getting a reasonable understanding about the role of biofilm control alone in the prevention/ control of dental caries. In most cases, toothbrushing is performed using fluoridated dentifrices and a great variety of fluoridated products are available for domiciliary use. These facts make it difficult to isolate the role of self-performed biofilm control in the conservative treatment of carious lesions, including those at root surfaces.

Mechanical Biofilm Control

Laboratory Studies

There are a few laboratory studies assessing the effect of biofilm control on the treatment of root carious lesions. Nyvad et al. [1] published the results of an in situ study testing the hypothesis that oral hygiene measures associated with topical fluoride was able to arrest the carious process and to reduce the ongoing mineral loss in active root lesions. Sound root surface specimens were inserted into the lower partial dentures of 18 healthy subjects, and the biofilm removal in these specimens was suppressed during 3 months, aiming at the development of carious lesions. Over the following 3 months, individuals allocated in the test group were instructed to brush the root specimens meticulously once a day with 1,100 ppm fluoride toothpaste, which was supplemented with two intra-oral topical application of 2% solution of sodium fluoride (NaF) for 2 min. Participants allocated in the control group performed no brushing and received no topical fluoride. This in situ study showed that the total mineral content of root lesions submitted to daily biofilm control and topical fluoride for 3 months remained unaltered, with no further detectable mineral loss. Additionally, an increase in the mineral content at the surface layer of the treated root lesions was observed. The authors concluded that the oral hygiene regime, composed of daily biofilm removal and topical fluoride, may arrest the lesion progression in carious root surfaces.

To the best of our knowledge, this is the unique in situ study available in the literature addressing this issue. On the contrary, there are some experimental in situ and in vivo studies that provide evidences supporting the effect of oral hygiene on enamel caries [2–4]. These studies show that the elimination of oral hygiene procedures lead to the development of non-cavitated enamel lesions [2] and that regular mechanical biofilm control resulted in no further mineral loss [3] and in clinical arrestment of the lesion [4].

Clinical Studies

Oral hygiene is critical in the caries control process; nevertheless, there are also clinical evidences showing the benefit of supplementing oral hygiene procedures with chemical agents to achieve root caries control [5]. A recent systematic review, which collected and analyzed the clinical evidence concerning the efficiency of noninvasive treatments for root caries, concluded that "root caries could be controlled at the population level by daily brushing with fluoride-containing toothpastes, whilst active decay may be inactivated using professional application of fluoride varnishes/ solutions or self-applied high-fluoride toothpaste [5]." Studies on coronal caries also showed that for most subjects, tooth-brushing performance may be insufficient to control caries when using a fluoride-free toothpaste [6–8].

Studies on root caries control often motivate patients to perform oral hygiene [5]. This emphasizes the importance of biofilm control in the management of root caries. In a series of 24 cases of root cavities, Nyvad and Fejerskov [9] demonstrated the possibility of arresting root cavities by means of oral hygiene and topical fluoride. Initially, the carious lesions were greasy, yellowish, or light brownish, with a soft aspect under light probing (active lesions). The ten adult patients included in the study received instruction on oral hygiene mainly focused on their root cavities. During the same appointment, patients performed supervised biofilm removal, and the lesion received an application of 2% NaF solution for 2 min which was repeated after 8 weeks. The domiciliary hygiene procedures consisted of two daily toothbrushing period with a 1,000 ppm F dentifrice. No other source of fluoride was applied during the experimental period and the aspect of lesions concerning texture, color, and surface structure were registered for 18 months. Biofilm and/or gingival trauma were detected rarely and, in these cases, adjustments on the domiciliary toothbrushing technique were performed. Gradual changes in the color and surface texture were observed over the inactivation process, with lesions becoming harder and darker, with smoother margins and contours.

In another study, the possibility of converting active root carious lesions into inactive lesions by a 12-month prophylactic program with emphasis on oral hygiene procedures was evaluated [10]. In this program, 15 caries-active individuals received intensive oral hygiene training on an individual basis in the first 3 months (3–7 visits). Professional cleaning and application of fluoride varnish were performed at 3-, 6-, and 9-month visits. After 12 months of intervention, the number of active lesions decreased from 99 to 46, which represents an inactivation rate of around 50%. The authors also found that the proportion of lesions becoming inactive was not similar among the different root surfaces. Root caries lesions located at buccal and lingual surfaces were more likely to arrest over the study period than those located at approximal surfaces. This finding emphasizes the importance of accessibility to biofilm control of every dental site on a regular basis aiming at lesion arrestment.

In addition to these studies that assessed specifically the effect of oral hygiene and fluoride on the arrestment of active root cavities, there is some evidence derived from the control groups of clinical trials comparing products. Recently, a controlled clinical trial by Zhang et al. [11] compared 3 strategies to prevent and arrest root caries among community-dwelling elders from Hong Kong: group 1 (the control group) received oral hygiene instructions (OHIs) annually; group 2 received OHI and silver diamine fluoride (SDF) application annually, and group 3 received OHI and SDF application annually, associated with an oral health education program every 6 months. After 24 months, 227 individuals were available for follow-up. It was observed that a higher mean number of active root lesions became inactive in groups 2 and 3 than in group 1, with groups 2 and 3 showing similar aspects for arrested lesions. This finding leads us to conclude that the SDF exerted an additional effect on caries arrestment compared to OHI only. With regard to caries prevention, group 3 showed a lower mean number of new root lesions than group 1, with no difference observed for group 2. It evidences that the beneficial effect of a well-structured oral health education program in addition to OHI + SDF (group 3) exceeded the benefits of OHI + SDF alone (group 2).

In another randomized clinical trial by Tan et al. [12], 203 elders were followed for 3 years to compare 4 different methods used in preventing new root lesions. Individuals receiving individualized OHI and a placebo solution every 3 months developed a higher number of new lesions than those who received OHI and applications of chlorhexidine varnish, NaF varnish, or SDF solu-

Table 1. Epidemiological studies evaluating the association between self-reported oral hygiene habits and root caries

Reference	Author (year)	Country	Sample	Main finding
Cross-sectional studies				
13	Vehkalahti et al. (1997)	Slovenia	410 26–74-year-olds	No statistically significant differences in root caries occurrence by different frequencies of toothbrushing
14	Imazato et al. (2006)	Japan	287 60–78-year-olds	Toothbrushing frequency neither associated with decayed root lesions nor with decayed/filled root lesions
18	Du et al. (2009)	China	1,080 35–44-year-olds 1,080 65–74-year-olds	% of individuals with RCI >0 significantly higher among those reporting a toothbrushing frequency of < once a day In risk assessment analysis, no association
15	Sugihara et al. (2010)	Japan	153 60–94-year-olds	No correlation between toothbrushing frequency and root caries
19	Hayes et al. (2016)	Ireland	334 ≥65-year-olds	Toothbrushing frequency (<once a day) significantly associated with RDFS >0 in the bivariate analysis. No association in the multivariate model Interdental cleaning not associated with RDFS >0 in both analysis
Longitudinal studies				
16	Gilbert et al. (2001)	USA	723 ≥45-year-olds at baseline	Toothbrushing frequency not significantly associated with increment of root caries over 24 months
17	Siukosaari et al. (2005)	Finland	71	Toothbrushing frequency not associated with RCI increment over 5 years

RCI, Root caries index; RDFS, root decayed and filled surfaces.

tion. All these experimental groups had significant protective effects against the development of new root lesions compared to the control group.

These clinical studies disclose the possibility of adopting a systematic biofilm control, aided by the use of chemical agents (different topical fluoride agents, chlorhexidine, arginine, and so on), as preventing programs and/or conservative treatments for root carious lesions.

Epidemiological Studies

The relationship between oral hygiene practices and root caries has also been investigated in epidemiological studies, as shown in Table 1. In general, despite different settings, sample sizes, and age groups, epidemiological studies are consistent in showing no significant association between self-reported toothbrushing frequency and the occurrence of root caries, both in cross-sectional [13–15] and longitudinal [16, 17] studies. Some studies found significant associations in preliminary analysis [18] or bivariate models [19], but when the variable "toothbrushing frequency" were included in multivariable/adjusted models, no significant association was observed.

The epidemiological surveys described in Table 1 adopted self-reported data, in which subjects spontaneously reported their oral hygiene habits by means of questionnaires or interviews. Considering the limitation of this information when compared to data generated by clinical examinations, the lack of association herein reported must be taken into perspective.

Although these epidemiological studies did not associate root caries with frequency of toothbrushing, Tan and Lo [20] found significant association between the presence of biofilm and decayed root surfaces.

The majority of epidemiological studies do not show association of dental biofilm with root caries. Due to the multifactorial nature of caries, the presence of dental biofilm does not imply caries development. Caries management should target the equilibrium between risk factors (such as sugar exposure and dental biofilm accumulation) and protective factors (such as fluoride exposure and salivary parameters).

Methods

Self-performed mechanical methods are the most cost-effective way to perform biofilm control on a daily basis. It involves several factors, such as knowledge on oral diseases and oral health instruction, manual dexterity, adequacy of cleaning instruments, patient commitment, and motivation.

Toothbrushing is the method of choice for cleaning free surfaces, with consistent evidences showing the effectiveness of toothbrushing in reducing the levels of dental biofilm [21] and in controlling dental caries when associated with fluoridated toothpaste [22]. End-tuft toothbrushes may be useful in cleaning specific sites where conventional toothbrushes hardly reach, including the furcation region of multi-rooted teeth and the bottom of cervical/root cavities.

Regarding the cleaning of approximal surfaces, the use of interdental brushes appears to be more effective than dental floss and wood sticks in the control of biofilm and gingivitis [23]. Notwithstanding, when there is no sufficient interdental space available, flossing remains the best available tool to perform interproximal cleaning. The literature suggests that self-performed dental flossing has limited additional effects as adjunct to toothbrushing for controlling interproximal caries [24, 25]. Although there is no study assessing its effectiveness on caries occurrence, the use of interdental brushes should be the first tool recommended for controlling approximal root cavities in patients with open interdental spaces considering its effectiveness on biofilm and gingivitis control.

It is important to emphasize that most studies available in the literature assessed the effect of different tools on the control of plaque and gingivitis, few studies used coronal caries as the outcome and none assessed specifically root caries.

Chemical Biofilm Control

Different chemical agents for supplement or even substitute mechanical biofilm control are commercially available. The chemical agent may be added to dentifrices or it may be provided through different vehicles, such as gels, varnishes, or mouth rinses. Since the focus of this chapter is to discuss oral hygiene practices, we will briefly discuss those agents available for home use (dentifrices and mouth rinses), with the exception of fluoridated products, discussed in the chapter by Magalhães, this volume, pp. 83–87.

Chlorhexidine digluconate for chemical biofilm control has been widely studied, and is available in several concentrations and vehicles. Mouth rinses in either alcohol-based (ethanol) or nonalcoholic formulations (0.12%) are widely recommended for biofilm control for periodontal purposes, but its effectiveness in caries control is still under debate. Two clinical trials assessed the effectiveness of chlorhexidine 0.12% solution in caries control among elders. Wyatt and MacEntee [26] showed that the daily use of chlorhexidine 0.12% mouth rinse was similar to a placebo solution. On the contrary, the other experimental group using a 0.2 neutral NaF solution had significantly less caries and more reversals of carious lesions to sound surfaces during the trial than the other groups. At the 2-year examination, the prevalence of root lesions was 80, 59, and 78% in groups using chlorhexidine, fluoride, and placebo solutions, respectively. The study by Wyatt et al. [27] followed individuals using chlorhexidine 0.12% solution or a placebo solution for 5 years. The authors performed a surface-level survival analysis and showed survival rates of 86% for root surfaces receiving chlorhexidine and 85% for root surfaces receiving the placebo solution. Powell et al. [28] also showed similar results following weekly 0.12% chlorhexidine rinses with or without fluoride varnish application twice a year in the occurrence of root caries events. In conjunction, these clinical trials suggest that regular rinsing with chlorhexidine has no substantial effect on caries control in older adults.

Triclosan is a chemical agent added to dentifrices in an attempt to improve the biofilm control. A systematic review assessed the effect of triclosan/copolymer-containing fluoridated toothpastes on the control of several oral outcomes, including caries [29]. According to the authors, only one study at high risk of bias showed a statistically significant reduction in root caries in favor of triclosan/copolymer after 36 months [30]. The review concluded that there is weak evidence to show that triclosan/copolymer toothpastes may reduce root caries.

In the last decade, the addiction of arginine to fluoridated dentifrices appeared as a biochemical alternative to the control of cariogenic challenge in the tooth-biofilm interface. Arginine is an amino acid that, when metabolized by the microorganisms of dental biofilm, provides the liberation of ammonia and a shift in the biofilm pH. A recent meta-analysis [5] revealed that dentifrices containing 1.5% arginine plus 1,400 ppm fluoride were more effective in arresting root caries than another product containing 1,100–1,400 ppm F alone. Notwithstanding, there is still room for controversy and the results presented to this date are being subject of questionings. The authors of another meta-analysis published in 2016 [31] suggest difficulties concerning the extrapolation of the results to other populations and possible bias due to the lack of methodological rigor and to the conflict of interest in some studies. According to the authors, more rigorous studies addressing the use of arginine as a supplement to fluoridated dentifrices are required.

The discovery of any supplement capable of enhancing the preventive properties of dentifrices is welcome by the dental community. This amino acid, naturally occurring in saliva and some foods, and presenting a biochemical activity plausible with the enhancement of the biofilm pH, appears to be promising. However, in the present date, its inclusion as an additive to dental care products is not unanimously accepted.

Conclusion

Oral hygiene is of utmost importance in the prevention of root caries. Whilst there is limited evidence on the control of dental caries solely by biofilm control, there is a wealth of evidence on the adjunctive effect of fluoride on the root caries control.

Active dental caries can be inactivated by means of biofilm control and topical fluoride. This approach is especially useful in lesions accessible to mechanical removal of biofilm, not dolorous and in cases where the aesthetic is not of primordial importance.

Traditionally, restorative treatment is an option to treat a cavitated carious lesion, mainly when aesthetic commitment and/or dolorous sensibility are present. The poor mechanical retention of root cavities, the limited long-term quality of the adhesion to dentin, and, in some situations, difficulties in moisture control are aspects to be considered during the treatment process. Furthermore, the indication of a filling to treat a root cavity will contribute to the restorative cycle, demanding filling repair or replacement over the life time, which notably reduces tooth longevity [32].

References

1 Nyvad B, ten Cate JM, Fejerskov O: Arrest of root surface caries in situ. J Dent Res 1997;76:1845–1853.
2 Von der Fehr FR, Löe H, Theilade E: Experimental caries in man. Caries Res 1970;4:131–148.
3 Dijkman A, Huizinga E, Ruben J, Arends J: Remineralization of human enamel in situ after 3 months: the effect of not brushing versus the effect of an F dentifrice and an F-free dentifrice. Caries Res 1990;24:263–266.
4 Holmen L, Thylstrup A, Artun J: Clinical and histological features observed during arrestment of active enamel carious lesions in vivo. Caries Res 1987;21:546–554.
5 Wierichs RJ, Meyer-Lueckel H: Systematic review on noninvasive treatment of root caries lesions. J Dent Res 2015;94:261–271.
6 Koch G, Lindhe J: The state of the gingivae and the caries-increment in schoolchildren during and after withdrawal of various prophylactic measures; in McHugh WD (ed): Dental Plaque. Edinburgh, Livingstone, 1970, pp 271–281.
7 Sutcliffe P: A longitudinal clinical study of oral cleanliness and dental caries in school children. Arch Oral Biol 1973;18:765–770.
8 Bellini HT, Arneberg P, von der Fehr FR: Oral hygiene and caries. A review. Acta Odontol Scand 1981;39:257–265.
9 Nyvad B, Fejerskov O: Active root surface caries converted into inactive caries as a response to oral hygiene. Scand J Dent Res 1986;94:281–284.
10 Emilson CG, Ravald N, Birkhed D: Effects of a 12-month prophylactic programme on selected oral bacterial populations on root surfaces with active and inactive carious lesions. Caries Res 1993;27:195–200.
11 Zhang W, McGrath C, Lo EC, Li JY: Silver diamine fluoride and education to prevent and arrest root caries among community-dwelling elders. Caries Res 2013;47:284–290.
12 Tan HP, Lo EC, Dyson JE, Luo Y, Corbet EF: A randomized trial on root caries prevention in elders. J Dent Res 2010;89:1086–1090.
13 Vehkalahti MM, Vrbic VL, Peric LM, Matvoz ES: Oral hygiene and root caries occurrence in Slovenian adults. Int Dent J 1997;47:26–31.
14 Imazato S, Ikebe K, Nokubi T, Ebisu S, Walls AW: Prevalence of root caries in a selected population of older adults in Japan. J Oral Rehabil 2006;33:137–143.
15 Sugihara N, Maki Y, Okawa Y, Hosaka M, Matsukubo T, Takaesu Y: Factors associated with root surface caries in elderly. Bull Tokyo Dent Coll 2010;51:23–30.
16 Gilbert GH, Duncan RP, Dolan TA, Foerster U: Twenty-four month incidence of root caries among a diverse group of adults. Caries Res 2001;35:366–375.
17 Siukosaari P, Ainamo A, Närhi TO: Level of education and incidence of caries in the elderly: a 5-year follow-up study. Gerodontology 2005;22:130–136.
18 Du M, Jiang H, Tai B, Zhou Y, Wu B, Bian Z: Root caries patterns and risk factors of middle-aged and elderly people in China. Community Dent Oral Epidemiol 2009;37:260–266.
19 Hayes M, Da Mata C, Cole M, McKenna G, Burke F, Allen PF: Risk indicators associated with root caries in independently living older adults. J Dent 2016;51:8–14.
20 Tan HP, Lo EC: Risk indicators for root caries in institutionalized elders. Community Dent Oral Epidemiol 2014;42:435–440.
21 Van der Weijden FA, Slot DE: Efficacy of homecare regimens for mechanical plaque removal in managing gingivitis a meta review. J Clin Periodontol 2015;42(suppl 16):S77–S91.
22 Marinho VC, Higgins JP, Sheiham A, Logan S: Fluoride toothpastes for preventing dental caries in children and adolescents. Cochrane Database Syst Rev 2003;1:CD002278. Review.
23 Sälzer S, Slot DE, Van der Weijden FA, Dörfer CE: Efficacy of inter-dental mechanical plaque control in managing gingivitis – a meta-review. J Clin Periodontol 2015;42(suppl 16):S92–S105.
24 Hujoel PP, Cunha-Cruz J, Banting DW, Loesche WJ: Dental flossing and interproximal caries: a systematic review. J Dent Res 2006;85:298–305.
25 Sambunjak D, Nickerson JW, Poklepovic T, Johnson TM, Imai P, Tugwell P, Worthington HV: Flossing for the management of periodontal diseases and dental caries in adults. Cochrane Database Syst Rev 2011;12:CD008829.
26 Wyatt CC, MacEntee MI: Caries management for institutionalized elders using fluoride and chlorhexidine mouthrinses. Community Dent Oral Epidemiol 2004;32:322–328.
27 Wyatt CC, Maupome G, Hujoel PP, MacEntee MI, Persson GR, Persson RE, Kiyak HA: Chlorhexidine and preservation of sound tooth structure in older adults. A placebo-controlled trial. Caries Res 2007;41:93–101.
28 Powell LV, Persson RE, Kiyak HA, Hujoel PP: Caries prevention in a community-dwelling older population. Caries Res 1999;33:333–339.
29 Riley P, Lamont T: Triclosan/copolymer containing toothpastes for oral health. Cochrane Database Syst Rev 2013;12:CD010514. Review.
30 Vered Y, Zini A, Mann J, DeVizio W, Stewart B, Zhang YP, Garcia L: Comparison of a dentifrice containing 0.243% sodium fluoride, 0.3% triclosan, and 2.0% copolymer in a silica base, and a dentifrice containing 0.243% sodium fluoride in a silica base: a three-year clinical trial of root caries and dental crowns among adults. J Clin Dent 2009;20:62–65.
31 Ástvaldsdóttir Á, Naimi-Akbar A, Davidson T, Brolund A, Lintamo L, Attergren Granath A, Tranæus S, Östlund P: Arginine and caries prevention: a systematic review. Caries Res 2016;50:383–393.
32 Elderton RJ: Preventive (evidence-based) approach to quality general dental care. Med Princ Pract 2003;12(suppl 1):12–21.

Marisa Maltz
Department of Social and Preventive Dentistry, Faculty of Odontology
Federal University of Rio Grande do Sul
Rua Ramiro Barcelos, 2492
Porto Alegre, RS 90035-003 (Brazil)
E-Mail marisa.maltz@gmail.com

Carrilho MRO (ed): Root Caries: From Prevalence to Therapy.
Monogr Oral Sci. Basel, Karger, 2017, vol 26, pp 83–87 (DOI: 10.1159/000479349)

Conventional Preventive Therapies (Fluoride) on Root Caries Lesions

Ana Carolina Magalhães

Department of Biological Sciences, Bauru School of Dentistry, University of São Paulo, Bauru, Brazil

Abstract

Root caries lesions (RCLs) are highly prevalent in elderly and can negatively impact the quality of life. Therefore, preventive therapies should be applied to control or to arrest RCLs. This chapter will discuss the application of fluoride, a conventional preventive therapy, to control RCLs. Among the self-applied products, there is strong evidence that 5,000 ppm F toothpaste is more effective in arresting RCLs (by increasing hardness) and in preventing new lesions (PF of 51%) compared to 1,100–1,450 ppm F toothpastes, in 6-month clinical trials. With regard to professional fluoride applications, 5% NaF varnish (4 times/year) and 38% silver diamine fluoride solution (1 time/year) have been tested in clinical trials with a follow-up of 3 years. Five percent NaF varnish and 38% silver diamine fluoride have been shown to prevent the emergence of new RCLs in 64 and 71%, respectively. The professional fluoride application is often combined with the daily use of 5,000 ppm F toothpaste. However, there is a gap in the knowledge about the benefit (cost-effectiveness) and the optimal use of the combinations of fluoride products in the control of RCLs.

Introduction

Currently, the generation of elderly is living longer than the past generations, and more than half of them have experience with root caries lesions (RCLs; Fig. 1), with a peak incidence around the age of 70 years and the estimated annual incidence of 23.3% [1, 2]. RCL is one of the causes of pain and tooth loss in elderly, with a negative impact on oral health-related quality of life [3]. Therefore, researchers and clinicians need to seek for an appropriate preventive approach to control the incidence and severity of RCLs in this population.

Fluoride has been widely applied for the prevention of dental caries, including RCLs [4]. Fluoride is known to reduce demineralization and improve remineralization. Further, it has some antimicrobial effect by reducing bacterial metabolism and interfering in proton extrusion [5]. However, most evidence on the effectiveness of fluoride in preventing dental caries is limited to populations of children (6–15 years old). With regard to RCLs, some evidence about the benefits of

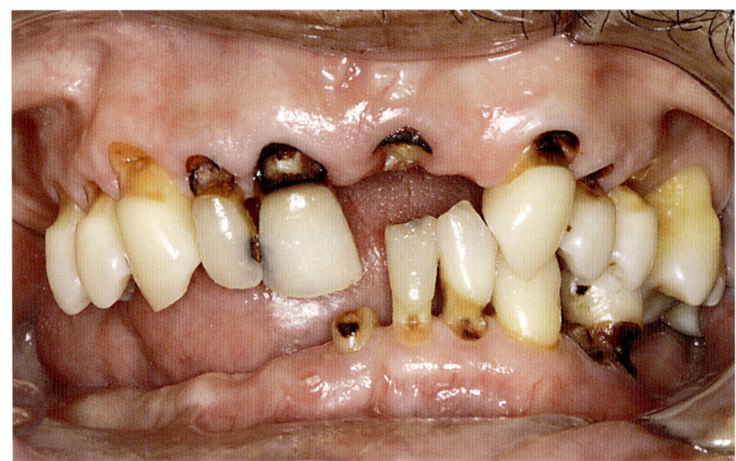

Fig. 1. Several root caries lesions found in a 60-year-old patient (photo taken by Marilia Velo, Marina Giacomini, Rafael Simões, Letícia Brianezzi and Linda Wang, Bauru School of Dentistry-USP, Brazil).

fluoride comes from clinical trials published in the last 10 years [6].

For this chapter, we selected recent clinical trials that compared different fluoride products and the association between them in preventing or arresting RCLs in elderly, with a follow-up between 6 months and 3 years. The most tested products containing fluoride are toothpastes, especially those containing 5,000 ppm F (applied twice a day), fluoride varnishes (5% NaF, applied every 3 months), and silver diamine fluoride solution (38%, applied once a year). Table 1 shows the results of some clinical trials discussed below.

Self-Applied Fluoride Products

Highly concentrated fluoride toothpastes (5,000 ppm F) have shown to significantly arrest RCLs (by hardness analysis) compared to conventional toothpastes containing 1,350–1,450 ppm F in clinical trials conducted during 6–8 months with elderly people, including disabled nursing home residents [7–9].

The application of 5,000 ppm F toothpaste, twice a day, is able to increase the fluoride concentration in saliva and biofilm as well as the formation of CaF_2 on tooth, and to reduce the biofilm formation and the level of *S. mutans* and *Lactobacillus* [10]. According to a systematic review, the relative risk for RCLs when 5,000 ppm F is compared to 1,100–1,450 ppm F is about 0.49, with a high level of evidence [11].

Some studies have also compared toothpaste containing 1.5% arginine and 1,450 ppm F with conventional 1,450 ppm F toothpaste, showing benefit of using fluoride toothpaste containing arginine in arresting and reversing RCLs [12, 13]. The main mechanism of action of arginine-based toothpastes is related to the formation of ammonia and the increase of biofilm pH [14]. According to a systematic review, the relative risk for RCLs when fluoride toothpaste containing arginine is compared to conventional fluoride toothpaste is about 0.79 [11]; however, in this case the level of evidence is very low [15].

Toothpastes or mouth rinses containing AmF/SnF_2 are able to decrease root caries initiation compared to NaF (standard mean differences, SMD = 0.15), but the evidence is low. Mouth rinses containing 225–900 ppm F^- as NaF were also revealed to reduce decayed, missing and filled root surfaces (DMFRS) compared to placebo (SMD = –0.18), but with a low level of evidence [11].

Based on the literature, there is no doubt that 5,000-ppm F toothpaste, applied twice a day during brushing, is the most evident choice for

Table 1. Results of some clinical trials on the effect of different fluoride products in preventing or arresting root caries in elderly or vulnerable adults

Authors	Number of subjects (age) Country	Fluoride products	Response variable Study duration	Main results
Souza et al. [12], 2013	253 (46) Brazil	1.5% arginine plus 1,450 vs. 1,450 ppm F toothpastes (twice a day)	ARC percentage 6 months	70.5 vs. 58.1% ($p < 0.05$)
Tan et al. [18], 2010	203 (79, institutionalized elderly) China	1% chlorhexidine (each 3 months) vs. 5% NaF varnish (each 3 months) vs. SDF (each year)	RC surface number 3 years	1.1 vs. 0.9 vs. 0.7 (ns)
Zhang et al. [16], 2013	227 (72.5) China	Oral hygiene instruction vs. OHI plus SDF (each year) vs. OHI plus SDF plus oral health education (each 6 months)	RC surface number/ ARC surface number 2 years	1.33[a] vs. 1.0[a, b] vs. 0.7[b]/0.04[a] vs. 0.28[b] vs. 0.33[b] ($p < 0.05$)
Ekstrand et al. [7], 2013	125 (82, disabled nursing home residents) Denmark	5,000 vs. 1,450 ppm F toothpastes (twice a day)	Active RC lesions number/ARC lesions number 8 months	1.05 vs. 2.55/2.13 vs. 0.61 ($p < 0.05$)
Srinivasan et al. [9], 2014	130 (57) Germany and Switzerland	5,000 vs. 1,350 ppm F toothpastes (twice a day)	Surface hardness improvement 6 months	2.4 vs. 2.8 ($p < 0.05$)
Li et al. [17], 2016	67 (72.2) China	SDF (each year, with or without PI) vs. control	ARC percentage 30 months	90 and 93% (with PI) vs. 45% ($p < 0.05$)
Xin et al. [22], 2016	78 (50, Sjögren's syndrome) China	5% NaF vs. placebo varnish (each 3 months)	RC surfaces and ARC surfaces 24 months	1.4 vs. 2.7 (ns) 0.3 vs. 0.1 (ns)

SDF, Silver diamine fluoride; OHI, oral hygiene instruction; ARC, arrested root caries; RC, root caries; PI, potassium iodide.

preventing and controlling RCLs. On the contrary, a range of clinical trials has also been conducted to test professional products for this purpose.

Professional-Applied Fluoride Products

Silver diamond fluoride solution/varnish and NaF varnish are the most often professional-applied products tested for RCL control. An annual application of 38% silver diamine fluoride has been shown to prevent and arrest RCLs in elderly people compared to education only, after 24–30 months of follow-up [16, 17]. Li et al. [17] showed that 90% of RCLs arrested after the application of silver diamine fluoride against 45% for the control group in a 30-month clinical trial.

The application of 1% chlorhexidine varnish, 5% NaF varnish (both each 3 months), and 38% silver diamine fluoride solution (once a year) was also compared for the prevention of RCLs in institutionalized elderly people [18]. Chlorhexidine, NaF, and silver diamine fluoride have shown to reduce in 56–57, 64, and 71–72% the development of new RCLs, respectively, with no significant differences observed after 3 years. According to the authors, silver diamine fluoride may be more advantageous when the frequency of application is considered [18]. Schwendicke and Göstemeyer [19] further showed that silver diamine fluoride (2×/year) might be a more cost-saving approach than NaF (daily mouth rinse application) or chlorhexidine (2×/year) in high-risk populations. Silver diamond fluoride has been also applied into prepared cavity lesions [20], reducing secondary root caries development around CIV restorations, with no evidence of affecting adhesion in vitro [21]. However, there is lack of clinical trials on this topic.

The major criticism with respect to silver diamond fluoride is that the precipitates oxidize, inducing tooth color alteration (dark color). However, the other products also present some limitations. Chlorhexidine can stain teeth and has a bitter taste. Fluoride varnish, depending on the brand name, can leave a yellow stain on the teeth for several hours after the application. Despite the disadvantages, patients usually accept all products.

A systematic review pointed out that the professional application of chlorhexidine or silver diamine fluoride varnish compared to placebo has significant impact on DMFRS (SMD = –0.33), but the evidence is still very low [11], due to the low number of well-conducted randomized controlled trials. The authors suggest that the regular use of toothpastes with 5,000 ppm F combined with annual applications of chlorhexidine or silver diamine fluoride should be indicated for the prevention of RCLs [11].

It is important to note that some factors have meaningful influence on the efficacy of fluoride on caries prevention. Elderly who wear any denture, with high visible plaque index scores, high baseline root caries experience, and great gingival recession develop more new RCLs over 3 years of follow up [16, 18].

Accordingly, the efficacy of fluoride on healthy elderly people cannot be translated to vulnerable adults with systemic diseases. Xin et al. [22] showed that fluoride varnish reduced only in 33% the number of carious dentin surfaces and slightly improve the remineralization compared to placebo in a 24-month clinical trial conducted with elderly presenting Sjogren's syndrome. Considering the lack of significant differences, this study did not provide clear evidence to support or reject the application of fluoride varnish for patients with Sjogren's syndrome.

Some authors prefer to combine the application of 5% NaF varnish (each 3 months) with the daily use of 5,000 ppm F toothpaste [23] as a protocol for preventing RCLs; while others have as primary approach the application of 38% silver diamine fluoride solution (1×/year) to prevent new RCLs and, as secondary, the application of 5% NaF varnish (each 3 months) to arrest RCLs, especially for vulnerable older adults [24]. Figure 2 shows a case of a patient with RCL, who was submitted to the F varnish treatment.

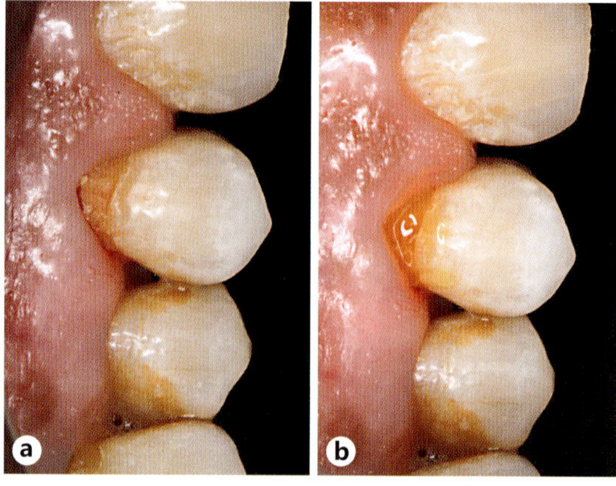

Fig. 2. a, b A case of root caries lesion (RCL) in a 60-year-old patient, who was previously under head and neck radiotherapy. The RCL was treated using fluoride varnish. The patient is under periodic control (photo taken by Marilia Velo, Marina Giacomini, Rafael Simões, Giovanna Zabeu, Letícia Brianezzi and Linda Wang, Bauru School of Dentistry-USP, Brazil).

Few studies were conducted to test fluoride mouth rinses, gels or foam on the prevention of RCLs and, in general, the quantity of evidence ranges from moderate (gel) to very low (foam) [25].

Conclusion

Despite some clinical evidence about the efficacy of fluoride on the prevention of RCLs (Table 1), there is a gap in the knowledge about the benefit (cost-effectiveness) and the optimal use of professional fluoride application combined with the daily use of fluoride toothpaste [25, 26]. Further well-designed clinical trials shall focus on the analysis of cost-effectiveness of fluoride combinations applied for preventing RCLs in both vulnerable adults and healthy elderly.

References

1 Griffin SO, Griffin PM, Swann JL, Zlobin N: Estimating rates of new root caries in older adults. J Dent Res 2004;83:634–638.
2 Liu L, Zhang Y, Wu W, Cheng M, Li Y, Cheng R: Prevalence and correlates of dental caries in an elderly population in northeast China. PLoS One 2013; 8:e78723.
3 Masood M, Newton T, Bakri NN, Khalid T, Masood Y: The relationship between oral health and oral health related quality of life among elderly people in United Kingdom. J Dent 2017;56:78–83.
4 Richards D: Fluoride has a beneficial effect on root caries. Evid Based Dent 2009;10:12.
5 Buzalaf MA, Pessan JP, Honório HM, ten Cate JM: Mechanisms of action of fluoride for caries control. Monogr Oral Sci 2011;22:97–114.
6 Griffin SO, Regnier E, Griffin PM, Huntley V: Effectiveness of fluoride in preventing caries in adults. J Dent Res 2007; 86:410–415.
7 Ekstrand KR, Poulsen JE, Hede B, Twetman S, Qvist V, Ellwood RP: A randomized clinical trial of the anti-caries efficacy of 5,000 compared to 1,450 ppm fluoridated toothpaste on root caries lesions in elderly disabled nursing home residents. Caries Res 2013;47:391–398.
8 Yeung CA: Some beneficial effect on root caries from use of higher concentration fluoride toothpaste (5000 ppm F). Evid Based Dent 2014;15:8–9.
9 Srinivasan M, Schimmel M, Riesen M, Ilgner A, Wicht MJ, Warncke M, et al: High-fluoride toothpaste: a multicenter randomized controlled trial in adults. Community Dent Oral Epidemiol 2014; 42:333–340.
10 Ekstrand KR: High fluoride dentifrices for elderly and vulnerable adults: does it Work and if so, then why? Caries Res 2016;50(suppl 1):15–21.
11 Wierichs RJ, Meyer-Lueckel H: Systematic review on noninvasive treatment of root caries lesions. J Dent Res 2015;94: 261–271.
12 Souza ML, Cury JA, Tenuta LM, Zhang YP, Mateo LR, Cummins D, et al: Comparing the efficacy of a dentifrice containing 1.5% arginine and 1450 ppm fluoride to a dentifrice containing 1450 ppm fluoride alone in the management of primary root caries. J Dent 2013; 41(suppl 2):S35–S41.
13 Hu DY, Yin W, Li X, Feng Y, Zhang YP, Cummins D, et al: A clinical investigation of the efficacy of a dentifrice containing 1.5% arginine and 1450 ppm fluoride, as sodium monofluorophosphate in a calcium base, on primary root caries. J Clin Dent 2013;24:A23–A31.
14 ten Cate JM, Cummins D: Fluoride toothpaste containing 1.5% arginine and insoluble calcium as a new standard of care in caries prevention. J Clin Dent 2013;24:79–87.
15 Li J, Huang Z, Mei L, Li G, Li H: Anticaries effect of arginine-containing formulations in vivo: a systematic review and meta-analysis. Caries Res 2015;49: 606–617.
16 Zhang W, McGrath C, Lo EC, Li JY: Silver diamine fluoride and education to prevent and arrest root caries among community-dwelling elders. Caries Res 2013;47:284–290.
17 Li R, Lo EC, Liu BY, Wong MC, Chu CH: Randomized clinical trial on arresting dental root caries through silver diammine fluoride applications in community-dwelling elders. J Dent 2016;51:15–20.
18 Tan HP, Lo EC, Dyson JE, Luo Y, Corbet EF: A randomized trial on root caries prevention in elders. J Dent Res 2010;89: 1086–1090.
19 Schwendicke F, Göstemeyer G: Cost-effectiveness of root caries preventive treatments. J Dent 2017;56:58–64.
20 Zhao IS, Mei ML, Burrow MF, Lo EC, Chu CH: Prevention of secondary caries using silver diamine fluoride treatment and casein phosphopeptide-amorphous calcium phosphate modified glass-ionomer cement. J Dent 2017;57:38–44.
21 Quock RL, Barros JA, Yang SW, Patel SA: Effect of silver diamine fluoride on microtensile bond strength to dentin. Oper Dent 2012;37:610–616.
22 Xin W, Leung KC, Lo EC, Mok MY, Leung MH: A randomized, double-blind, placebo-controlled clinical trial of fluoride varnish in preventing dental caries of Sjögren's syndrome patients. BMC Oral Health 2016;16:102.
23 Gibson G, Jurasic MM, Wehler CJ, Jones JA: Supplemental fluoride use for moderate and high caries risk adults: a systematic review. J Public Health Dent 2011;71:171–184.
24 Gluzman R, Katz RV, Frey BJ, McGowan R: Prevention of root caries: a literature review of primary and secondary preventive agents. Spec Care Dentist 2013; 33:133–140.
25 Twetman S, Keller MK: Fluoride rinses, gels and foams: an update of controlled clinical trials. Caries Res 2016;50(suppl 1):38–44.
26 Tellez M, Wolff MS: The public health reach of high fluoride vehicles: examples of innovative approaches. Caries Res 2016;50(suppl 1):61–67.

Ana Carolina Magalhães
Department of Biological Sciences, Bauru School of Dentistry, University of São Paulo
Al. Octávio Pinheiro Brisolla, 9-75
Bauru, SP 17012-901 (Brazil)
E-Mail acm@fob.usp.br

Carrilho MRO (ed): Root Caries: From Prevalence to Therapy.
Monogr Oral Sci. Basel, Karger, 2017, vol 26, pp 88–96 (DOI: 10.1159/000479350)

New Preventive Approaches Part I: Functional Peptides and Other Therapies to Prevent Tooth Demineralization

Marília Afonso Rabelo Buzalaf[a] • Juliano Pelim Pessan[b]

[a]Department of Biological Sciences, Bauru School of Dentistry, University of São Paulo, Bauru, and [b]Department of Pediatric Dentistry and Public Health, School of Dentistry, Araçatuba, São Paulo State University (Unesp), Araçatuba, Brazil

Abstract

The limited effect of fluoride on root caries has prompted the study of new preventive therapies, which involve recently developed functional peptides, lasers, phosphate-based technologies, among several other approaches. Most of the specific peptides currently investigated have been developed based on the available information related to the protective action of salivary proteins, including statherin-derived peptides. Other peptides include 8DSS, self-assembling peptide P11-4, antimicrobial peptides, and casein phosphopeptides combined with amorphous calcium phosphate. These were shown to increase remineralization and/or to protect against demineralization through different mechanisms, including the attraction of calcium ions to the demineralized tissue, delivery of available calcium, and antimicrobial action. Regarding phosphate-based technologies, the addition of polyphosphate salts to fluoridated vehicles has been shown to promote a synergistic effect in promoting enamel remineralization and in preventing demineralization, in studies with in vitro, in situ, and clinical protocols. Sodium trimetaphosphate has also been shown to promote intrafibrillar collagen remineralization, phosphate uptake by previously demineralized dentin, and deposition of needle-like crystallites at intrafibrillar level. As for the use of lasers, their effects on the mineral content and crystallinity of dentin were shown to be related to the removal of water and protein, besides surface melting by thermal degradation. Lasers have also been shown to have synergistic/additive effects with fluoride on the prevention of root dentin demineralization, due to the enhanced fluoride uptake and the decreased calcium and phosphate loss. Although the above-mentioned therapies seem to be promising alternatives to prevent root caries, clinical evidence is still required.

Introduction

The therapies available to fight root caries are less studied than those involving management of coronal caries. Similar to what has been reported for coronal caries, fluoride (F) is the most used agent for controlling root caries (for review, see the chapter by Burrow and Stacey, this volume, pp. 106–114), especially when high concentrations are employed [1]. A recent systematic review revealed that the regular use of dentifrices

Table 1. Salivary proteins related to protection against dental caries

Protein	Main finding	Reference
Albumin	Bovine serum albumin influences demineralization kinetics of hydroxyapatite in vitro	Kosoric et al. [82], 2010
Amylase	High concentration of amylase in unstimulated whole saliva protects against root caries in situ	Bardow et al. [80], 2005
Cystatin	Cystatin S and SN were present in higher concentrations in saliva and acquired pellicle of caries-free volunteers	Vitorino et al. [8], 2006
	Cystatin S was present in higher concentration in parotid saliva of elderly patients with root caries in comparison with controls	Preza et al. [83], 2009
	Cystatin B was increased in the acquired enamel pellicle after exposure to lactic acid in vivo	Delecrode et al. [5], 2015
Hystatin	Large amount of hystatin 1 in saliva of caries-free volunteers	Vitorino et al. [6], 2005
Mucin	Significant negative correlation between MUC5B and the number of decayed teeth in school children	Angwaravong et al. [9], 2015
	Addition of mucin (577 mg/L) in demineralization solution reduces mineral loss and lesion depth in vitro	Kielbassa et al. [81], 2005
PRPs	Large amounts of IB-7, a peptide resulting from cleavage of basic PRPs in saliva of caries-free subjects	Ayad et al. [7], 2000
	Large amounts of PRP1/3 in saliva of caries-free volunteers	Vitorino et al. [6], 2005
	Acidic PRPs were present in higher concentrations in saliva and acquired pellicle of caries-free volunteers	Vitorino et al. [8], 2006
Statherin	Large amounts of statherin in saliva of caries-free volunteers	Vitorino et al. [6], 2005

PRPs, Proline-rich proteins.

containing 5,000 ppm F and quarterly professionally applied chlorhexidine or F varnishes seem to be efficacious in decreasing the progression and initiation of root caries, respectively. However, this conclusion is based on very few well-conducted randomized controlled trials [2].

In addition to the use of fluoride, new preventive therapies have been proposed to prevent root demineralization, which involve recently developed functional peptides and other therapies, such as phosphate-based strategies and lasers. Some of these new proposed therapies will be discussed in this chapter.

Functional Peptides

Saliva is the most important host factor affecting the progression of dental caries. Several characteristics and properties of saliva play an important role in dental caries, such as salivary clearance, buffering capacity, and supersaturation with respect to tooth mineral. In addition, many proteins in saliva and acquired pellicle are involved in dental caries [3, 4], although most of the studies refer to enamel caries (Table 1). The early pellicle proteins, proline-rich proteins, and statherin, promote remineralization by attracting calcium ions [4], whereas acid-resistant proteins, such as cystatins, might reduce demineralization [5]. In addition, several proteins prevent the adherence of oral microorganisms to the acquired pellicle and inhibit their growth, while others are involved in the first line of defense in the oral cavity [4]. Clinical studies comparing the salivary protein composition of caries-free versus caries-susceptible subjects, revealed larger quantities of phosphopeptides (PRP1/3, histatin 1, and statherin) [6] and of a peptide (IB-7) resulting from cleavage of basic PRPs [7], as well as of PRP1/2 and protease inhibitors such as lipocalin and cystatins S and SN [8] in saliva from the caries-free group when compared with the caries-susceptible one. In addition, a significant negative correlation was found between MUC5B and the number of decayed teeth in school children [9]. Thus, most of the specific peptides currently investigated to protect against caries have been developed based on the available information related to the protective action of salivary proteins. However, considering the actual knowledge regarding the role of salivary proteins in protecting against demineralization (Table 1), there are many other peptides derived from salivary proteins that should be developed and evaluated.

Specific Peptides

The studies involving the development of specific peptides to protect against caries have all been conducted with enamel. These studies are in an initial stage of development and, in general, clinical data are not available yet. Among them, some evaluated the use of peptides derived from statherin [10, 11], a 43-residue phosphorylated protein. Its negative charge density and helical conformation at the N-terminus are important for the interaction with hydroxyapatite [12]. Solid-state nuclear magnetic resonance studies confirmed that the N-terminus of statherin strongly binds to hydroxyapatite, while the middle and C-terminal regions are mobile and dynamic [13]. It has been shown in vitro that statherin-derived peptides containing at least 15 N-terminal residues (StN21 and StN15) are required for binding to hydroxyapatite and reducing demineralization [11]. However, there are studies neither conducted with dentin nor using protocols that more closely resemble the clinical condition.

Peptides derived from enamel and dentin proteins have also been developed. Among them is 8DSS, constituted of octuplet repeats of aspartate-serine-serine derived from dentin phosphoprotein that are believed to nucleate the formation of hydroxyapatite [14]. 8DSS promoted mineral deposition over demineralized enamel surfaces, improving its mechanical properties [15]. Moreover, it was able to remineralize initial enamel caries [16] and to inhibit enamel demineralization in vitro, having a synergistic effect with fluoride [16]. Similar to what has been reported for statherin-derived peptides, studies on dentin or using more clinically relevant protocols are not available so far.

A self-assembling peptide (P11-4) has also been suggested to increase remineralization and inhibit demineralization [17]. When applied on the white spot lesion, P11-4 penetrates into the pores due to its low viscosity and triggers self-assembly within the lesion, forming negatively charged fibers that attract calcium ions, thus nucleating hydroxyapatite mineral [18]. In vitro experiments have reported enamel remineralization after the application of P11-4 [17, 19, 20]. Moreover, single application of P11-4 was shown to improve the appearance of white spot lesions after 180 days in a small-scale clinical study [18]. However, more evidence is still necessary before this peptide can be used in caries prevention and therapy. Studies involving root dentin are also desired.

Some peptides, known as antimicrobial peptides (AMPs), are able to provide the early stage of protection against invading microbes, being promising substitutes for conventional antibiotics. They are short, cationic host-defense molecules that have important modulatory roles and act as a bridge between innate and acquired immunity [21]. Synthetic peptides, designed to minimize mutans streptococci counts in the oral cavity (thus having a role against caries) have been developed. These are called specifically targeted antimicrobial peptides (STAMPs) [22]. A plethora of peptides have been evaluated mostly in vitro and shown to be effective against mutans streptococci, as well as to avoid enamel demineralization in situ (for review, see references [21], [23] and [24]). Despite these successes, current peptides can be unstable and expensive to produce. In addition, it is also extremely difficult to extrapolate in vitro results to in vivo microenvironments during drug discovery phases [24]. A recent study showed that salivary concentrations of individual AMPs were not associated with the severity of early childhood caries. However, combination of different AMPs was positively associated with caries levels [25]. Although the anticaries potential of AMPs and STAMPs has been extensively evaluated, mainly in vitro, but also in situ, clinical studies evaluating their role on caries progression are not available so far. In addition, the effect of the combination of different AMPs and/or STAMPs could be evaluated to allow the development of an effective product. It must be highlighted that studies evaluating their effect against root caries are not available in the literature.

Casein phosphopeptides (CPP) combined with amorphous calcium phosphate (ACP), known as CPP-ACP technology or Recaldent™, have also been used to prevent caries. In the oral cavity, CPP-ACP can act at enamel and dentin, where ACP binds to hydroxyapatite. Furthermore, CPP-ACP can diffuse into dental biofilm and protect tooth surfaces against demineralization by (1) presenting a buffering capacity (which neutralizes the pH after a cariogenic challenge); (2) increasing biofilm calcium concentrations; and (3) localizing ACP in the biofilm [26]. Although most of the animal, in vitro and in situ studies (for review, see [27]), including those conducted with dentin [28–31], report a good potential of CPP-ACP to reduce demineralization and to enhance remineralization, systematic reviews of clinical trials highlight lack of good quality evidence to make conclusions regarding the long-term effectiveness of CPP-ACP in preventing caries in vivo [32–34]. High-quality, well-designed clinical studies in this area are still required before definitive recommendations can be made.

Phosphate-Based Strategies

Considering the limited effects of fluoride on the de- and remineralization processes of tooth structures, there has been an increasing interest on phosphate-based strategies, used alone or in combination with fluoride in oral care products. Polyphosphate salts, nano-hydroxyapatite particles, calcium glycerophosphate, amorphous calcium phosphate (please see above under "functional peptides"), and functionalized β-tricalcium phosphate are some examples of the technologies that have been mostly investigated over recent years. This review will focus on some polyphosphates and calcium glycerophosphate.

Polyphosphates

There has been an increasing interest in the study of polyphosphate salts as additives to fluoride in a variety of vehicles for topical application. Among these, sodium trimetaphosphate (TMP) and sodium hexametaphosphate (HMP) are cyclic polyphosphates that have been shown to promote synergistic effects against hydroxyapatite dissolution [35, 36], reducing enamel demineralization [37–40], enhancing enamel remineralization [41–43], and reducing enamel erosive wear [44–46], using in vitro and in situ protocols. Such effects have been recently confirmed in a randomized clinical trial, in which the rate of caries progression in children using a low-F toothpaste containing TMP was significantly lower than that observed for children brushing with a conventional formulation (1,110 ppm F) without TMP [47].

The largest body of evidence is available for TMP in a variety of vehicles including rinses, gels, varnishes, toothpastes, in studies showing synergistic preventive and therapeutic effects between fluoride and TMP depending on the appropriate molar ratio in the formulation. Such synergism was observed in toothpastes with fluoride concentrations as low as 250 μg F/g, which reached a protective effect similar to the conventional formulation (1,100 μg F/g) [48]. Such effects were further enhanced by the use of nanosized TMP, with a marked effect on the subsurface lesion and variables related to the biofilm [49].

Despite containing phosphate in their structure, these salts cannot be considered as a source of free phosphate to react with the tooth structures (enamel and dentin), given that their cyclic molecules do not become spontaneously hydrolyzed under physiological conditions [50, 51]. Instead, the effect of these salts is related to their ability to interact with the tooth surfaces: in the oral environment, these salts become negatively charged (due to the release of Na^+ ions), allowing binding to Ca^{2+} in the outermost layers, thus forming a protective layer that limits acid diffusion and enhances calcium and fluoride diffusion into enamel. In this sense, it has been proposed that such protective layer is able to retain fluoride compounds that are released upon cariogenic challenges, leading to the formation of more reactive compounds [42], similar to CPP-ACP [52].

While most of the studies on the effects of TMP and HMP were performed with tooth enamel, there is some evidence that these salts also present therapeutic properties on dentin. TMP was shown to promote the phosphorylation of type I collagen in demineralized dentin [53], and to induce intrafibrillar collagen remineralization [54] (please see the chapter by Burrow and Stacey, this volume, pp. 106–114 for collagen modifiers). Also, the application of a self-etching primer doped with TMP and an adhesive containing calcium and phosphate nanofillers was shown to decrease nanoleakage within the resin-dentin interfaces, besides promoting phosphate uptake by previously demineralized dentin, and deposition of needle-like crystallites at intrafibrillar level [55]. The above-mentioned studies taken together seem to indicate that therapies involving TMP might be an effective strategy for the prevention of root caries, so that future studies in this field would be instructive.

Calcium Glycerophosphate

Similarly as described for TMP, calcium glycerophosphate (CaGP) has been studied as an additive to fluoridated toothpastes to enhance their preventive and therapeutic effects on dental caries. The addition of CaGP to low-fluoride toothpastes (500–550 ppm F) promoted a similar anticaries effect when compared to a 1100 ppm F toothpaste, considering enamel remineralization in situ [56], enamel demineralization in vitro [57] and in situ [58], biofilm fluoride concentrations [58], and caries progression in children, in a randomized clinical trial [47]. Also, salivary fluoride concentrations were shown to be significantly increased when CaGP was administered prior to fluoride [59]. Studies with different protocols, however, failed to demonstrate a synergistic effect between fluoride and CaGP in toothpastes [60] and varnishes [61]. As for TMP, an appropriate fluoride:CaGP molar ratio is paramount for achieving optimum results.

The possible mechanisms of action seem to be related to interactions with enamel during de- and remineralization processes similar to TMP, in addition to elevated fluoride, calcium, and phosphate levels in the biofilm, plaque-pH buffering, and direct interaction with dental mineral [56, 58, 62]. Regarding the protective effects on dentin demineralization, in vitro evidence shows a dose-response relationship between CaGP concentration and dentin mineral loss only when this salt was applied prior to a cariogenic challenge [62]. Although the effects of CaGP associated with fluoride on dentin have not yet been studied, the evidence available for enamel suggest that the addition of CaGP to fluoridated products might be another strategy for the prevention of root caries.

Lasers

The application of lasers on dental hard tissues (enamel and dentin) has been shown to promote preventive effects on dental caries when used with sub-ablative energies [63]. A substantial number of in vitro studies have been conducted for over 4 decades, attempting to reduce enamel acid dissolution. CO_2 lasers at wavelength of 9.6 or 9.3 μm, short pulsed at the microsecond range, have been intensively studied for caries prevention [64]; other laser wavelengths have also been investigated, including Nd:YAG, Er:YAG, Er,Cr:YSGG, and argon lasers [65]. The effects of laser therapies may vary according to the type of dental tissue, level of energy applied, wavelength, and pulse time.

The ability of lasers to modify the properties of enamel surface are related to the irradiation heat on the enamel surface at a temperature below enamel melting, what promotes loss of the carbonate phase from the enamel crystals which, in turn, reduces enamel acid dissolution [64, 65]. Regarding dentin, the effects of laser irradiation on the mineral content and crystallinity were shown to be related to the removal of water and protein [66], besides surface melting by thermal degradation [63]. Despite the high temperatures achieved at the outermost enamel or dentin surfaces, there is evidence that there is no harm to the pulpal tissue [67, 68].

Most of the laboratory studies have described a synergistic or additive effect of topical fluoride application and laser therapy on the prevention of demineralization of root dentin. The application of Er,Cr:YSGG [69] or CO_2 [70] lasers associated with 2% NaF gel was shown to increase acid resistance of human root dentin in vitro, similar to what was observed for CO_2 laser in association with 1,23% APF (acidulated phosphate fluoride) gel [71] or 5% NaF fluoride varnish [68], or Er:YAG laser in combination with silver diamine fluoride [72]. Such synergistic effects seem to be related to the enhanced fluoride uptake by dentin [70], as well as to the decreased loss of calcium and phosphate [71] promoted by the laser. Using an in situ protocol, however, no additive benefit was verified for irradiation with CO_2 and application of 1,23% APF gel [73], suggesting that intraoral variables not included in in vitro studies may also play a role in the clinical outcome. Irradiation with CO_2 laser has also been shown to significantly reduce dentin mineral loss around composite resin restorations in vitro [74, 75], but not for specimens restored with a fluoride-releasing material (glass ionomer cement) [75].

Evidence from the few in vivo studies conducted to date are consistent with most of the laboratory data described above, showing significant reductions in enamel smooth surface mineral loss around orthodontic brackets after irradiation with CO_2 laser only [76], and argon [77] or Nd:YAG [78] lasers associated with fluoride. Similar findings were also reported for fissures of permanent molars in association with a 5% NaF varnish compared with varnish alone [65]. For dentin root caries, no clinical study has yet been conducted. However, based on (1) the promising in vitro and in situ data obtained for dentin regarding acid resistance, and (2) the favorable clinical evidence for the treatment of dentin hypersensitivity [79], the use of laser therapy, especially in association with topical fluoride, seems to be a promising alternative for the control of root caries.

In conclusion, some of the therapies not involving fluorides that have been recently developed to prevent root demineralization involve functional peptides, phosphate-based strategies, and lasers. Although these therapies seem to be promising alternatives to prevent root caries, clinical evidence is still required before they can be broadly used.

References

1 Petersson LG: The role of fluoride in the preventive management of dentin hypersensitivity and root caries. Clin Oral Investig 2013;17(suppl 1):S63–S71.
2 Wierichs RJ, Meyer-Lueckel H: Systematic review on noninvasive treatment of root caries lesions. J Dent Res 2015;94: 261–271.
3 Buzalaf MA, Hannas AR, Kato MT: Saliva and dental erosion. J Appl Oral Sci 2012;20:493–502.
4 Van Nieuw Amerongen A, Bolscher JG, Veerman EC: Salivary proteins: protective and diagnostic value in cariology? Caries Res 2004;38:247–253.
5 Delecrode TR, Siqueira WL, Zaidan FC, Bellini MR, Moffa EB, Mussi MC, et al: Identification of acid-resistant proteins in acquired enamel pellicle. J Dent 2015; 43:1470–1475.
6 Vitorino R, Lobo MJ, Duarte JR, Ferrer-Correia AJ, Domingues PM, Amado FM: The role of salivary peptides in dental caries. Biomed Chromatogr 2005;19: 214–222.
7 Ayad M, Van Wuyckhuyse BC, Minaguchi K, Raubertas RF, Bedi GS, Billings RJ, et al: The association of basic proline-rich peptides from human parotid gland secretions with caries experience. J Dent Res 2000;79:976–982.
8 Vitorino R, de Morais Guedes S, Ferreira R, Lobo MJ, Duarte J, Ferrer-Correia AJ, et al: Two-dimensional electrophoresis study of in vitro pellicle formation and dental caries susceptibility. Eur J Oral Sci 2006;114:147–153.
9 Angwaravong O, Pitiphat W, Bolscher JG, Chaiyarit P: Evaluation of salivary mucins in children with deciduous and mixed dentition: comparative analysis between high and low caries-risk groups. Clin Oral Investig 2015;19: 1931–1937.
10 Santos O, Kosoric J, Hector MP, Anderson P, Lindh L: Adsorption behavior of statherin and a statherin peptide onto hydroxyapatite and silica surfaces by in situ ellipsometry. J Colloid Interface Sci 2008;318:175–182.
11 Shah S, Kosoric J, Hector MP, Anderson P: An in vitro scanning microradiography study of the reduction in hydroxyapatite demineralization rate by statherin-like peptides as a function of increasing N-terminal length. Eur J Oral Sci 2011;119(suppl 1):13–18.
12 Raj PA, Johnsson M, Levine MJ, Nancollas GH: Salivary statherin. Dependence on sequence, charge, hydrogen bonding potency, and helical conformation for adsorption to hydroxyapatite and inhibition of mineralization. J Biol Chem 1992;267:5968–5976.
13 Naganagowda GA, Gururaja TL, Levine MJ: Delineation of conformational preferences in human salivary statherin by 1H, 31P NMR and CD studies: sequential assignment and structure-function correlations. J Biomol Struct Dyn 1998; 16:91–107.
14 George A, Bannon L, Sabsay B, Dillon JW, Malone J, Veis A, et al: The carboxyl-terminal domain of phosphophoryn contains unique extended triplet amino acid repeat sequences forming ordered carboxyl-phosphate interaction ridges that may be essential in the biomineralization process. J Biol Chem 1996;271: 32869–32873.
15 Hsu CC, Chung HY, Yang JM, Shi W, Wu B: Influence of 8DSS peptide on nano-mechanical behavior of human enamel. J Dent Res 2011;90:88–92.
16 Yang Y, Lv XP, Shi W, Li JY, Li DX, Zhou XD, et al: 8DSS-promoted remineralization of initial enamel caries in vitro. J Dent Res 2014;93:520–524.
17 Kirkham J, Firth A, Vernals D, Boden N, Robinson C, Shore RC, et al: Self-assembling peptide scaffolds promote enamel remineralization. J Dent Res 2007;86: 426–430.
18 Brunton PA, Davies RP, Burke JL, Smith A, Aggeli A, Brookes SJ, et al: Treatment of early caries lesions using biomimetic self-assembling peptides – a clinical safety trial. Br Dent J 2013;215:E6.
19 Jablonski-Momeni A, Heinzel-Gutenbrunner M: Efficacy of the self-assembling peptide P11-4 in constructing a remineralization scaffold on artificially-induced enamel lesions on smooth surfaces. J Orofac Orthop 2014;75:175–190.
20 Schmidlin P, Zobrist K, Attin T, Wegehaupt F: In vitro re-hardening of artificial enamel caries lesions using enamel matrix proteins or self-assembling peptides. J Appl Oral Sci 2016;24:31–36.
21 Mai S, Mauger MT, Niu LN, Barnes JB, Kao S, Bergeron BE, et al: Potential applications of antimicrobial peptides and their mimics in combating caries and pulpal infections. Acta Biomat 2017;49: 16–35.
22 Eckert R, He J, Yarbrough DK, Qi F, Anderson MH, Shi W: Targeted killing of Streptococcus mutans by a pheromone-guided "smart" antimicrobial peptide. Antimicrob Agents Chemother 2006;50: 3651–3657.
23 Eckert R, Sullivan R, Shi W: Targeted antimicrobial treatment to re-establish a healthy microbial flora for long-term protection. Adv Dent Res 2012;24:94–97.
24 Pepperney A, Chikindas ML: Antibacterial peptides: opportunities for the prevention and treatment of dental caries. Probiotics Antimicrob Proteins 2011;3: 68.
25 Colombo NH, Ribas LF, Pereira JA, Kreling PF, Kressirer CA, Tanner AC, et al: Antimicrobial peptides in saliva of children with severe early childhood caries. Arch Oral Biol 2016;69:40–46.
26 Nongonierma AB, Fitzgerald RJ: Biofunctional properties of caseinophosphopeptides in the oral cavity. Caries Res 2012;46:234–267.
27 Reynolds EC: Casein phosphopeptide-amorphous calcium phosphate: the scientific evidence. Adv Dent Res 2009;21: 25–29.
28 Mazzaoui SA, Burrow MF, Tyas MJ, Dashper SG, Eakins D, Reynolds EC: Incorporation of casein phosphopeptide-amorphous calcium phosphate into a glass-ionomer cement. J Dent Res 2003;82:914–918.
29 Oshiro M, Yamaguchi K, Takamizawa T, Inage H, Watanabe T, Irokawa A, et al: Effect of CPP-ACP paste on tooth mineralization: an FE-SEM study. J Oral Sci 2007;49:115–120.
30 Rahiotis C, Vougiouklakis G: Effect of a CPP-ACP agent on the demineralization and remineralization of dentine in vitro. J Dent 2007;35:695–698.
31 Yamaguchi K, Miyazaki M, Takamizawa T, Inage H, Kurokawa H: Ultrasonic determination of the effect of casein phosphopeptide-amorphous calcium phosphate paste on the demineralization of bovine dentin. Caries Res 2007;41: 204–207.
32 Azarpazhooh A, Limeback H: Clinical efficacy of casein derivatives: a systematic review of the literature. J Am Dent Assoc 2008;139:915–924.

33 Li J, Xie X, Wang Y, Yin W, Antoun JS, Farella M, et al: Long-term remineralizing effect of casein phosphopeptide-amorphous calcium phosphate (CPP-ACP) on early caries lesions in vivo: a systematic review. J Dent 2014;42:769–777.

34 Yengopal V, Mickenautsch S: Caries preventive effect of casein phosphopeptide-amorphous calcium phosphate (CPP-ACP): a meta-analysis. Acta Odontol Scand 2009;67:321–332.

35 do Amaral JG, Delbem ACB, Pessan JP, Manarelli MM, Barbour ME: Effects of polyphosphates and fluoride on hydroxyapatite dissolution: a pH-stat investigation. Arch Oral Biol 2016;63:40–46.

36 Manarelli MM, Pessan JP, Delbem AC, Amaral JG, Paiva MF, Barbour ME: Protective effect of phosphates and fluoride on the dissolution of hydroxyapatite and their interactions with saliva. Caries Res 2017;51:96–101.

37 Takeshita EM, Castro LP, Sassaki KT, Delbem AC: In vitro evaluation of dentifrice with low fluoride content supplemented with trimetaphosphate. Caries Res 2009;43:50–56.

38 Takeshita EM, Danelon M, Castro LP, Sassaki KT, Delbem AC: Effectiveness of a toothpaste with low fluoride content combined with trimetaphosphate on dental biofilm and enamel demineralization in situ. Caries Res 2015;49:394–400.

39 da Camara DM, Pessan JP, Francati TM, Santos Souza JA, Danelon M, Delbem AC: Synergistic effect of fluoride and sodium hexametaphosphate in toothpaste on enamel demineralization in situ. J Dent 2015;43:1249–1254.

40 da Camara DM, Pessan JP, Francati TM, Souza JA, Danelon M, Delbem AC: Fluoride toothpaste supplemented with sodium hexametaphosphate reduces enamel demineralization in vitro. Clin Oral Investig 2016;20:1981–1985.

41 Danelon M, Takeshita EM, Sassaki KT, Delbem AC: In situ evaluation of a low fluoride concentration gel with sodium trimetaphosphate in enamel remineralization. Am J Dent 2013;26:15–20.

42 Manarelli MM, Delbem AC, Lima TM, Castilho FC, Pessan JP: In vitro remineralizing effect of fluoride varnishes containing sodium trimetaphosphate. Caries Res 2014;48:299–305.

43 Manarelli MM, Delbem AC, Binhardi TD, Pessan JP: In situ remineralizing effect of fluoride varnishes containing sodium trimetaphosphate. Clin Oral Investig 2015;19:2141–2146.

44 Moretto MJ, Delbem AC, Manarelli MM, Pessan JP, Martinhon CC: Effect of fluoride varnish supplemented with sodium trimetaphosphate on enamel erosion and abrasion: an in situ/ex vivo study. J Dent 2013;41:1302–1306.

45 Conceição JM, Delbem AC, Danelon M, da Camara DM, Wiegand A, Pessan JP: Fluoride gel supplemented with sodium hexametaphosphate reduces enamel erosive wear in situ. J Dent 2015;43:1255–1260.

46 Cruz NV, Pessan JP, Manarelli MM, Souza MD, Delbem AC: In vitro effect of low-fluoride toothpastes containing sodium trimetaphosphate on enamel erosion. Arch Oral Biol 2015;60:1231–1236.

47 Freire IR, Pessan JP, Amaral JG, Martinhon CC, Cunha RF, Delbem AC: Anti-caries effect of low-fluoride dentifrices with phosphates in children: a randomized, controlled trial. J Dent 2016;50:37–42.

48 Missel EM, Cunha RF, Vieira AE, Cruz NV, Castilho FC, Delbem AC: Sodium trimetaphosphate enhances the effect of 250 p.p.m. fluoride toothpaste against enamel demineralization in vitro. Eur J Oral Sci 2016;124:343–348.

49 Souza MDB, Pessan JP, Lodi CS, Souza JAS, Camargo ER, Souza Neto FN, Delbem ACB: Toothpaste with nano-sized trimetaphosphate reduces enamel demineralization. JDR Clin Trans Res 2017, in press.

50 Castellini E, Lusvardi G, Malavasi G, Menabue L: Thermodynamic aspects of the adsorption of hexametaphosphate on kaolinite. J Colloid Interface Sci 2005;292:322–329.

51 Choi IK, Wen WW, Smith RW: Technical note the effect of a long chain phosphate on the adsorption of collectors on kaolinite. Miner Eng 1993;6:1191–1197.

52 Cochrane NJ, Saranathan S, Cai F, Cross KJ, Reynolds EC: Enamel subsurface lesion remineralisation with casein phosphopeptide stabilised solutions of calcium, phosphate and fluoride. Caries Res 2008;42:88–97.

53 Zhang X, Neoh KG, Lin CC, Kishen A: Remineralization of partially demineralized dentine substrate based on a biomimetic strategy. J Mater Sci Mater Med 2012;23:733–742.

54 Sauro S, Osorio R, Watson TF, Toledano M: Influence of phosphoproteins' biomimetic analogs on remineralization of mineral-depleted resin-dentin interfaces created with ion-releasing resin-based systems. Dent Mater 2015;31:759–777.

55 Abuna G, Feitosa VP, Correr AB, Cama G, Giannini M, Sinhoreti MA, Pashley DH, Sauro S: Bonding performance of experimental bioactive/biomimetic self-etch adhesives doped with calcium-phosphate fillers and biomimetic analogs of phosphoproteins. J Dent 2016;52:79–86.

56 Zaze AC, Dias AP, Amaral JG, Miyasaki ML, Sassaki KT, Delbem AC: In situ evaluation of low-fluoride toothpastes associated to calcium glycerophosphate on enamel remineralization. J Dent 2014;42:1621–1625.

57 Zaze AC, Dias AP, Sassaki KT, Delbem AC: The effects of low-fluoride toothpaste supplemented with calcium glycerophosphate on enamel demineralization. Clin Oral Investig 2014;18:1619–1624.

58 do Amaral JG, Sassaki KT, Martinhon CC, Delbem AC: Effect of low-fluoride dentifrices supplemented with calcium glycerophosphate on enamel demineralization in situ. Am J Dent 2013;26:75–80.

59 Vogel GL, Shim D, Schumacher GE, Carey CM, Chow LC, Takagi S: Salivary fluoride from fluoride dentifrices or rinses after use of a calcium pre-rinse or calcium dentifrice. Caries Res 2006;40:449–454.

60 Tenuta LM, Cenci MS, Cury AA, Pereira-Cenci T, Tabchoury CP, Moi GP, Cury JA: Effect of a calcium glycerophosphate fluoride dentifrice formulation on enamel demineralization in situ. Am J Dent 2009;22:278–282.

61 Carvalho TS, Peters BG, Rios D, Magalhães AC, Sampaio FC, Buzalaf MA, Bönecker MJ: Fluoride varnishes with calcium glycerophosphate: fluoride release and effect on in vitro enamel demineralization. Braz Oral Res 2015;29:pii:S1806-83242015000100287.

62 Lynch RJ, ten Cate JM: Effect of calcium glycerophosphate on demineralization in an in vitro biofilm model. Caries Res 2006;40:142–147.

63 Rodrigues JA, Lussi A, Seemann R, Neuhaus KW: Prevention of crown and root caries in adults. Periodontol 2000 2011;55:231–249.

64 Tassery H, Levallois B, Terrer E, Manton DJ, Otsuki M, Koubi S, Gugnani N, Panayotov I, Jacquot B, Cuisinier F, Rechmann P: Use of new minimum intervention dentistry technologies in caries management. Aust Dent J 2013;58(suppl 1):40–59.
65 Rechmann P, Charland DA, Rechmann BM, Le CQ, Featherstone JD: In-vivo occlusal caries prevention by pulsed CO2-laser and fluoride varnish treatment – a clinical pilot study. Lasers Surg Med 2013;45:302–310.
66 Fried D, Zuerlein MJ, Le CQ, Featherstone JD: Thermal and chemical modification of dentin by 9-11-microm CO2 laser pulses of 5-100-micros duration. Lasers Surg Med 2002;31:275–282.
67 Goodis HE, Fried D, Gansky S, Rechmann P, Featherstone JD: Pulpal safety of 9.6 microm TEA CO2 laser used for caries prevention. Lasers Surg Med 2004;35:104–110.
68 Esteves-Oliveira M, El-Sayed KF, Dörfer C, Schwendicke F: Impact of combined CO_2 laser irradiation and fluoride on enamel and dentin biofilm-induced mineral loss. Clin Oral Investig 2017;21: 1243–1250.
69 Geraldo-Martins VR, Lepri CP, Faraoni-Romano JJ, Palma-Dibb RG: The combined use of Er,Cr:YSGG laser and fluoride to prevent root dentin demineralization. J Appl Oral Sci 2014; 22:459–464.
70 Gao XL, Pan JS, Hsu CY: Laser-fluoride effect on root demineralization. J Dent Res 2006;85:919–923.
71 Esteves-Oliveira M, Zezell DM, Ana PA, Yekta SS, Lampert F, Eduardo CP: Dentine caries inhibition through CO(2) laser (10.6μm) irradiation and fluoride application, in vitro. Arch Oral Biol 2011;56:533–539.
72 Mei ML, Ito L, Chu CH, Lo EC, Zhang CF: Prevention of dentine caries using silver diamine fluoride application followed by Er:YAG laser irradiation: an in vitro study. Lasers Med Sci 2014;29: 1785–1791.
73 Colucci V, Messias DC, Serra MC, Corona SA, Turssi CP: Fluoride plus CO2 laser against the progression of caries in root dentin. Am J Dent 2012;25:114–117.
74 de Melo JB, Hanashiro FS, Steagall W Jr, Turbino ML, Nobre-dos-Santos M, Youssef MN, de Souza-Zaroni WC: Effect of CO2 laser on root caries inhibition around composite restorations: an in vitro study. Lasers Med Sci 2014;29: 525–535.
75 Daniel LC, Araújo FC, Zancopé BR, Hanashiro FS, Nobre-dos-Santos M, Youssef MN, Souza-Zaroni WC: Effect of a CO_2 laser on the inhibition of root surface caries adjacent to restorations of glass ionomer cement or composite resin: an in vitro study. ScientificWorldJournal 2015;2015:298575.
76 Rechmann P, Fried D, Le CQ, Nelson G, Rapozo-Hilo M, Rechmann BM, Featherstone JD: Caries inhibition in vital teeth using 9.6-μm CO2-laser irradiation. J Biomed Opt 2011;16:071405.
77 Hicks J, Winn D 2nd, Flaitz C, Powell L: In vivo caries formation in enamel following argon laser irradiation and combined fluoride and argon laser treatment: a clinical pilot study. Quintessence Int 2004;35:15–20.
78 Zezell DM, Boari HG, Ana PA, Eduardo Cde P, Powell GL: Nd:YAG laser in caries prevention: a clinical trial. Lasers Surg Med 2009;41:31–35.
79 Bal MV, Keskiner İ, Sezer U, Açıkel C, Saygun I: Comparison of low level laser and arginine-calcium carbonate alone or combination in the treatment of dentin hypersensitivity: a randomized split-mouth clinical study. Photomed Laser Surg 2015;33:200–205.
80 Bardow A, Hofer E, Nyvad B, ten Cate JM, Kirkeby S, Moe D, et al: Effect of saliva composition on experimental root caries. Caries Res 2005;39:71–77.
81 Kielbassa AM, Oeschger U, Schulte-Monting J, Meyer-Lueckel H: Microradiographic study on the effects of salivary proteins on in vitro demineralization of bovine enamel. J Oral Rehabil 2005;32:90–96.
82 Kosoric J, Hector MP, Anderson P: The influence of proteins on demineralization kinetics of hydroxyapatite aggregates. J Biomed Mater Res A 2010;94: 972–977.
83 Preza D, Thiede B, Olsen I, Grinde B: The proteome of the human parotid gland secretion in elderly with and without root caries. Acta Odontol Scand 2009;67:161–169.

Prof. Marília Afonso Rabelo Buzalaf
Department of Biological Sciences, Bauru School of Dentistry, University of São Paulo
Al. Octávio Pinheiro Brisolla, 9-75
Bauru, SP 17012-901 (Brazil)
E-Mail mbuzalaf@fob.usp.br

Carrilho MRO (ed): Root Caries: From Prevalence to Therapy.
Monogr Oral Sci. Basel, Karger, 2017, vol 26, pp 97–105 (DOI: 10.1159/000479351)

New Preventive Approaches Part II: Role of Dentin Biomodifiers in Caries Progression

Ana K. Bedran-Russo • Camila A. Zamperini

Department of Restorative Dentistry, University of Illinois at Chicago, Chicago, IL, USA

Abstract

Dental caries is the most prevalent infectious chronic disease in children and adults. With a globally aging population, new demands in the management of dental caries are awakened by the rampant increase in the incidence of dental root caries. Like crown caries, root caries requires bacterial driven tissue demineralization followed by the degradation of the extracellular dentin matrix. Due to the complex composition and ultrastructure, preventive strategies targeting the mineral phase of dentin are insufficient for managing the prevention and progression of root caries. However, the composition and ultrastructure of dentin has inspired novel strategies for the effective management of highly susceptible root surfaces. Specifically, the complex and dynamic dentin extracellular matrix (ECM). The ECM of mature dentin contains a robust type I collagen fibrils scaffold, and carefully distributed non-collagenous components, such as proteoglycans, phosphoproteins, and proteases. In this chapter, we will review the experimental strategies of potential clinical impact to prevent root caries progression by site modifications of the mature extracellular dentin matrix. This approach, termed *dentin biomodification*, encompasses bioinspired strategies to locally enhance the biological and biomechanical characteristics of the tissue by mimicking natural processes. Here, synthetic and biosynthetic compounds can decrease the biodegradability of the dentin ECM and provide mechanical enhancement of dentin. The resulting effect is the maintenance of the dentin ECM to halt root caries progression and possibly mediate effective remineralization of the caries affected root dentin.

Introduction

Similar to crown dentin caries, the root caries progression involves 2 events: (a) the mineral content (from cementum and/or dentin) is dissolved as a result of repetitive imbalances between acidic byproducts from dental biofilms and pH compensatory mechanisms from oral cavity (de-remineralization balance) [1], and (b) the dentin extracellular organic matrix is susceptible to degradation. The degradation of the extracellular matrix (ECM) plays a critical role in the progression of the dentin caries. Particularly, the solubilization of type I collagen, the main component of the dentin ECM. Host-derived enzymes activated in the process of caries formation can degrade dentin collagen [2–

4]. Endogenous matrix metalloproteinase and cysteine cathepsins in dentin, saliva, and dentinal fluid [2, 3, 5–10] play a key role in the dentin matrix degradation, as discussed in the chapter by Boukpessi et al., this volume, pp. 35–42.

Role of the ECM on Root Caries Progression and Remineralization

Although the demineralization was for a long time a simplistic way of understanding the progression of caries, the role of the dentin organic matrix has gained increased attention. Several investigations have focused on determining the mechanisms implicated in the degradation of the dentin ECM [5, 11, 12]. In a balanced de-remineralization scenario (healthy condition), the dentin collagen fibrils are fully impregnated by extra- and intrafibrillar minerals facilitated by non-collagenous proteins, such as proteoglycans and phosphoproteins. During the initial demineralization, the extrafibrillar mineral content (e.g., mineral present between collagen fibrils) is dissolved more quickly than the intrafibrillar mineral content (e.g., mineral present within the collagen fibrils, preferentially in the gap zone between collagen molecules); increasing the intrafibrillar relative mineral concentration [13]. The maintenance of intrafibrillar minerals within the gap zones of the collagen fibrils is of fundamental importance for the remineralization of apatite nucleation sites (nucleation dependent-remineralization) and for the recovery of dentin mechanical properties [13–16].

Ideally, the intrafibrillar remineralization is followed by extrafibrillar remineralization for the complete enveloping of the collagen network [16]. Thus, the dentin organic matrix functions as an essential collagenous scaffold for the mineral uptake and growth that ideally leads to successful functional remineralization including the complete recovery of mechanical properties. Sustaining a sound extracellular cellular matrix is key for re-establishing the matrix-mineral ratio for the recovery of mechanical properties and ultimately the dentin function [13–16].

ECM Components Relevant to Dentin Biomodification

There are 4 ECM components of particular interest for utilizing dentin biomodification strategies for the root caries management: type I collagen, proteoglycans, phosphoproteins, and endogenous proteases. In this chapter, we will provide a brief overview on these key components.

Fibrillar Type I Collagen

Type I collagen comprises 90% of total organic content in dentin. It is a strong and elastic biomaterial arranged in highly organized hierarchical structures [17]. The collagen fibrils are formed by spontaneous self-assembly of the molecules into a periodic structure with 67–69 nm repeat period overlap between neighboring molecules, which is crucial for the development of covalent intermolecular cross-linking. The intermolecular cross-linking is the final post-translational modification of collagen, and is the basis for the stability, tensile strength, and viscoelasticity of collagen fibrils.

The slope of the elastic stress-strain curve for collagen increases with increased degree of cross-linking [18], so that there is a positive correlation between enzymatically induced collagen cross-linking and mechanical properties of the collagen-based tissue. Subtle perturbations to the cross-linking profile have been correlated with detrimental effects to the strength of mineralized tissue, such as bone and dentin [19]. In addition, the biodegradability and thermal stability of the tissue is also controlled by the amount and type of collagen cross-linking. Endogenous collagen cross-linkings are mediated by enzymatic and non-enzymatic reactions. Enzymatic intra- and intermolecular cross-links are formed between telopeptides and adjacent triple helical chains through lysine-lysine covalent bonding [20, 21].

Non-enzymatic collagen cross-linkings are mostly mediated by oxidation and glycation processes [22]. Exogenous collagen cross-linking can be induced by non-enzymatic reaction sources such as chemical and physical agents, and they have varying mechanism of interaction with type I collagen.

Proteoglycans
Dentin proteoglycans are a major group of non-collagenous components identified in both pre-dentin and dentin. Small leucine-rich proteoglycans play a crucial role in dentin biomineralization and in the structural integrity of collagen fibrils [23]. In addition to their roles in biomineralization, proteoglycans control tissue hydration and molecule diffusivity [24]. Thus, proteoglycans regulate the mechanical behavior of the dentin by controlling water displacement within intra- and intertubular dentin. Modified forms of the tissue, such as sclerotic dentin, can affect the PGs distribution [25].

Dentin Phosphoproteins
Dentin phosphoproteins are involved in the maturation of mineralized dentin, binding large amounts of calcium and modulating the dentin crystal growth. Dentin phosphoproteins are the most abundant non-collagenous proteins in dentin [26] with varying distribution between dentin and pre-dentin. There is still poor understanding of the presence and distribution profile of these proteins and their regulatory role in the remineralization process of natural carious dentin.

Endogenous Proteases
Endogenous proteases such as matrix metalloproteinases (MMPs) can degrade different components of the ECM. In the oral cavity, MMPs are involved in the progression of periodontal disease, caries (detailed in the chapter by Boukpessi et al., this volume, pp. 35–42), pulp inflammation, and oral cancer [2, 27, 28]. In the dentin-pulp complex, several MMPs have been identified, such as MMP-2, -3, -8, and -9 [29–31]. Another important family of proteases are the cysteine cathepsins [32, 33]. Cathepsins are active in acidic pH, and participate in the ECM degradation in physiological and pathological biological processes. In addition to their role in caries progression [32] (detailed in the chapter by Boukpessi et al., this volume, pp. 35–42), cathepsins have also been associated with other oral diseases, such as periodontitis, bone resorption, and oral cancer. Like MMPs, cathepsins are active in intact and carious dentin and show decreased activity with age.

Biomodification of Dentin – A Bioinspired Strategy

The biomodification of mature hard tissues, specifically dentin, is a novel bioinspired strategy to locally improve the biostability and function of the tissue for preventive or reparative/restorative purposes. Such strategies primarily target type I collagen due to its key role in dentin biomineralization. The approach was initially thought to be driven only by inter- or intramolecular collagen-induced non-enzymatic collagen cross-linking [34]. However, multi-interactions between certain bioactive agents with various dentin components result in additional desirable effects, such as protease inhibition and changes in tissue hydrophilicity. Ultimately, the physicochemical changes of the mature dentin will directly affect the local tissue biomechanics and biodegradability.

Types and Sources of Dentin Biomodifiers
Well-known synthetic agents, nature-derived agents, and also physical methods have been shown to effectively interact with type I collagen. The sources and types of biomodification agents are classified in a similar manner as collagen cross-linking agents. A brief overview of agents with known effect on dentin is described below and in Figure 1.

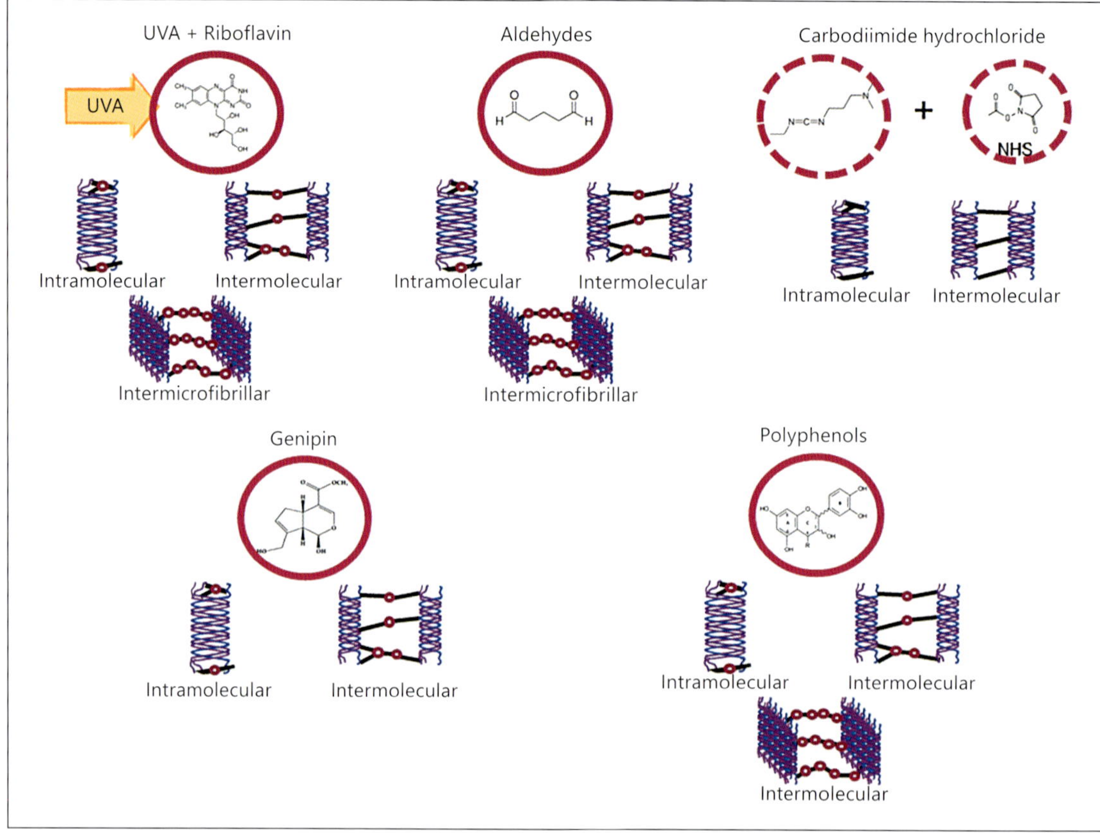

Fig. 1. Schematic drawing of the dentin biomodification agents and their mechanism of interactions with type I collagen. Agents are represented by red circles. Except for carbodiimide, all other agents are part of the newly formed exogenous collagen cross-linking.

Synthetic Collagen Biomodifiers

Synthetic collagen modifiers can mediate collagen cross-linking either by physical methods or by chemical agents. Physical methods utilize photo-oxidation method, more frequently by light exposure, especially ultraviolet radiation [35, 36]. The photo-oxidative method requires the presence of singlet oxygen; and riboflavin (vitamin B2) is one of the most potent producers of these oxygen radicals [37]. Photo-activation of riboflavin results in singlet-oxygen-inducing chemical covalent bonds, bridging amine groups (N-H) of glycine of one chain with carbonyl groups (C = O) of hydroxyproline and proline in adjacent chains [38]. Photo-activation of riboflavin with UVA is effective [39]; however, there are safety concerns with the use and clinical applicability of UVA.

The use of *synthetic chemical compounds* encompasses the largest selection of potential synthetic agents. Aldehydes are well studied compounds that cross-link collagen, with glutaraldehyde being the most widely known agent of this class. Glutaraldehyde is a dialdehyde with high affinity for active nitrogen groups of amino acids [40] and reacts primarily with the ε-amino groups of peptidyl lysine and hydroxylysine residues of collagen fibrils. Glutaraldehyde has been shown to decrease the rates of collagen degradation [41] and enhance the mechanical properties of dentin ECM [42]. A major disadvantage of this agent is the high cytotoxicity [43] and its residual effect, limiting clinical applicability. Glutaraldehyde is present in few dental products as a desensitizer and antimicrobial. Formaldehyde and triglyceraldehydes are examples of other aldehydes with similar cross-linking mechanism.

Carbodiimide Hydrochloride (EDC)
EDC is as a "zero-length" agent due to its ability to cross-link peptides in collagen without introducing additional linkage groups. EDC cross-links collagen by the activation of carboxylic acid groups of glutamic and aspartic acids to form an O-acylisourea intermediate. The latter reacts with the ε-amino groups of lysine or hydroxylysine to form an amide cross-link. Urea is formed as a by-product of the final cross-linking reaction that can be readily removed from the tissue. The use of N-hydroxysuccinimide is effective in increasing the number of induced collagen cross-linking and preventing the hydrolysis of activated carboxyl groups [44, 45]. While the cross-linking potential is limited [46], EDC are less toxic than aldehydes [47]. In addition, the inhibitory effect of EDC on endogenous and exogenous enzymatic activities is well documented [46, 48].

Biosynthetic Collagen Biomodifiers
In the past decades, naturally occurring collagen biomodifiers have received great attention in dentistry. Many of the natural compounds have been investigated for many decades as anti-microbial agents for caries prevention [34, 49]. One of their most attractive characteristics is their low toxicity when compared to synthetic agents [43] and their extensive use as dietary supplements.

Genipin
Genipin is an iridoid compound that interacts with collagen by inducing intramolecular cross-linking by reactions with free amino acid (lysine, hydroxylysine, or arginine) to form a nitrogen iridoid that undergoes dehydration to form an aromatic monomer [50, 51]. A downside is their slow collagen cross-linking reaction and deep blue staining of the tissue, thus limiting clinical applications.

Polyphenols
Polyphenols represent secondary plant metabolites divided into classes of polyphenolic compounds: phenolic acids, flavonoids (sub-classes: flavones, isoflavones, flavanols, flavanones, and anthocyanins), stilbenes, and lignans [52]. An important aspect of flavonoid chemistry is the formation of oligomers/polymers from monomers such as epicatechin or quercetin by mutual condensation, or conjugation with sugars [53] and other phenolic acids such as gallic acid by condensation reactions (e.g., epigallocatechin gallate in green tea). The conjugated/condensed products are often confused with the monomers in their nomenclature and structure. One example is hesperidin, a flavanone glycoside derived from a glycone hesperetin; with the only difference between the 2 compounds being the presence of a disaccharide.

Of particular interest to dental application are flavonoids proanthocyanidins (PACs). PACs are divided into different classes based on the hydroxylation patterns in the A and B rings of the flavonoid skeleton. PACs containing (–) epicatechin (majority) or (+) catechin as their building blocks are known as procyanidins. The monomeric building blocks of PACs are flavan-3-ol units composed of 3 rings. The variability of monomeric compounds, their degree of polymerization, and structure chirality imparts an exceptional amount of structural diversity and complexity to the already complicated combinatorial chemistry of PACs [34].

The highly hydroxylated structure of PACs enables the formation of insoluble complexes with carbohydrates and proteins [54]. PACs and collagen form complexes stabilized primarily by hydrogen bonding between the protein amide carbonyl and the phenolic hydroxyl [55] and covalent [56]

Table 1. Summary of experimental outcomes of dentin biomodification agents on root caries

Authors, year	Study model	Cross-linking agents	Evaluation methods	Main findings
Xie et al. [65]	In vitro (pH cycling)	Proanthocyanidin-rich grape seed extract (6.5%)	Microhardness and polarized light and confocal laser scanning (CLSM) microscopies	Enhanced remineralization
Walter et al. [63]	In vitro (bacterial model)	Proanthocyanidin (0.5%), genipin (0.625%) and glutaraldehyde (5%)	SDS-PAGE and hydroxyproline analysis (biochemical tests); pH measurements and CLSM	Enhanced remineralization
Pavan et al. [66]	In vitro (pH cycling)	Proanthocyanidin-rich grape seed extract (6.5%)	Transverse microradiography (TMR)	Inhibited demineralization
Hiraishi et al. [67]	In vitro (pH cycling + bacterial collagenase)	Hesperidin (10, 100, 1,000 and 10,000 ppm)	Atomic absorption (calcium release determination), hydroxylproline assay, and TMR	Inhibited demineralization and enhanced remineralization
Epasinghe et al. [68]	In vitro (pH cycling)	Proanthocyanidin (6.5%)	Microhardness, TMR and CLSM	Enhanced remineralization
Epasinghe et al. [68]	In vitro (pH cycling)	Proanthocyanidin (6.5%), naringin (6.5%) and quercetin (6.5%)	Microhardness, TMR, and CLSM	Enhanced remineralization
Epasinghe et al. [69]	In vitro (pH cycling + bacterial collagenase)	Proanthocyanidin (6.5%)	TMR, CLSM, XRD spectra (crystal formation), hydroxylproline assay	Inhibited demineralization and enhanced remineralization
Kim et al. [64]	In vitro (bacterial model)	Proanthocyanidin (6.5%), carbodiimide	Fluorescent microscopy	Inhibited secondary caries around resin composite margins in root dentin

and hydrophobic pockets [43]. The relatively large stability of PACs-protein complex suggests structure specificity [57]. The strong inhibition of proteolytic activity and its effect on proteoglycans have broadened their dental applications [34]. Since PACs have multi-functionality [58–60], their effectiveness in the root caries therapy is multi-factorial as follow: (1) mediates reinforcement of the dentin collagen; (2) inhibits protease activity, and (3) functions as a non-collagenous proteins analog.

Experimental Effectiveness of Collagen Biomodifiers

Bioinspired strategies for caries management target the stability and function of the ECM to prevent and reduce root caries progression. To date, the effects of dentin biomodifiers on the root caries inhibition and remineralization have been largely experimentally investigated. The effectiveness of the dentin biomodification agents is believed to be due to the mediation of exogenous collagen cross-linkings of caries and sound dentin matrix [58, 60–62] and the inhibition of caries-related proteases, including MMPs (-2, -8, -9) and cysteine cathepsins (B and K) [59, 60]. These effects result in increased biostability of the dentin matrix. Table 1 summarizes some of the critical findings.

Under a bacterial model, glutaraldehyde and PACs have been shown to reduce root caries progression [63]. Also under a bacterial model, secondary caries around margins of restorations in root surfaces could be reduced by use of primers containing proanthocyanidins, but not carbodiimide [64]. Under a pH cycling model of artificial caries, the effectiveness of proanthocyanidin on the root caries inhibition is well documented [63,

65–69]. Comparatively, the PACs showed greater preventive effect on root lesion development than genipin and glutaraldehyde (positive control). PACs also exhibited greater MMPs and cysteine cathepsins inactivation than chlorhexidine [59].

Polyphenols are the most investigated dentin biomodifiers for caries prevention, because of their multi-interaction with the dentin ECM components. PACs can reduce the biodegradability of the extracellular dentin matrix [63], inactivate proteases (endogenous and exogenous) [5, 59], and promote remineralization by calcium nucleation (acting as a phosphoprotein analog) [65]. Other flavonoids, including naringin, quercetin, and hesperidin, also present beneficial effects on the stabilization of root caries collagen matrix [67, 68]. Similar to proanthocyanidin, they inhibited the demineralization and promoted the remineralization of artificial root caries lesions, and their effects were attributed to the ability of stabilizing the dentin matrix through mimicking hierarchical levels of collagen cross-linking.

Conclusion

Dentin biomodification agents are multi-functional biomaterials targeting components of the ECM of dentin. The primary mechanism of action of collagen biomodifiers in the root caries management is the biological reinforcement of the dentin ECM by direct interactions with dentin collagen. Selective agents have shown promising ability to induce remineralization as a calcium nucleator. In vivo studies are needed to determine the clinical effectiveness and applicability of the most promising agents on the root caries progression.

References

1 Takahashi N, Nyvad B: Ecological hypothesis of dentin and root caries. Caries Res 2016;50:422–431.
2 Tjaderhane L, Larjava H, Sorsa T, Uitto VJ, Larmas M, Salo T: The activation and function of host matrix metalloproteinases in dentin matrix breakdown in caries lesions. J Dent Res 1998;77:1622–1629.
3 Sulkala M, Wahlgren J, Larmas M, Sorsa T, Teronen O, Salo T, et al: The effects of MMP inhibitors on human salivary MMP activity and caries progression in rats. J Dent Res 2001;80:1545–1549.
4 Nishitani Y, Yoshiyama M, Wadgaonkar B, Breschi L, Mannello F, Mazzoni A, et al: Activation of gelatinolytic/collagenolytic activity in dentin by self-etching adhesives. Eur J Oral Sci 2006;114:160–166.
5 Vidal CM, Tjaderhane L, Scaffa PM, Tersariol IL, Pashley D, Nader HB, et al: Abundance of MMPs and cysteine cathepsins in caries-affected dentin. J Dent Res 2014;93:269–274.
6 Boushell LW, Kaku M, Mochida Y, Bagnell R, Yamauchi M: Immunohistochemical localization of matrixmetalloproteinase-2 in human coronal dentin. Arch Oral Biol 2008;53:109–116.
7 Shimada Y, Ichinose S, Sadr A, Burrow MF, Tagami J: Localization of matrix metalloproteinases (MMPs-2, 8, 9 and 20) in normal and carious dentine. Aust Dent J 2009;54:347–354.
8 Toledano M, Nieto-Aguilar R, Osorio R, Campos A, Osorio E, Tay FR, et al: Differential expression of matrix metalloproteinase-2 in human coronal and radicular sound and carious dentine. J Dent 2010;38:635–640.
9 Nascimento FD, Minciotti CL, Geraldeli S, Carrilho MR, Pashley DH, Tay FR, et al: Cysteine cathepsins in human carious dentin. J Dent Res 2011;90:506–511.
10 Charadram N, Farahani RM, Harty D, Rathsam C, Swain MV, Hunter N: Regulation of reactionary dentin formation by odontoblasts in response to polymicrobial invasion of dentin matrix. Bone 2012;50:265–275.
11 Deyhle H, Bunk O, Muller B: Nanostructure of healthy and caries-affected human teeth. Nanomedicine 2011;7:694–701.
12 Tjäderhane L, Buzalaf MA, Carrilho M, Chaussain C: Matrix metalloproteinases and other matrix proteinases in relation to cariology: the era of "dentin degradomics." Caries Res 2015;49:193–208.
13 Balooch M, Habelitz S, Kinney JH, Marshall SJ, Marshall GW: Mechanical properties of mineralized collagen fibrils as influenced by demineralization. J Struct Biol 2008;162:404–410.
14 Kinney JH, Habelitz S, Marshall SJ, Marshall GW: The importance of intrafibrillar mineralization of collagen on the mechanical properties of dentin. J Dent Res 2003;82:957–961.
15 Bertassoni LE, Habelitz S, Kinney JH, Marshall SJ, Marshall GW Jr: Biomechanical perspective on the remineralization of dentin. Caries Res 2009;43:70–77.
16 Bertassoni LE, Habelitz S, Marshall SJ, Marshall GW: Mechanical recovery of dentin following remineralization in vitro – an indentation study. J Biomech 2011;44:176–181.
17 Ortiz C, Boyce MC: Materials science. Bioinspired structural materials. Science 2008;319:1053–1054.
18 Silver FH, Horvath I, Foran DJ: Viscoelasticity of the vessel wall: the role of collagen and elastic fibers. Crit Rev Biomed Eng 2001;29:279–301.
19 Knott L, Bailey AJ: Collagen cross-links in mineralizing tissues: a review of their chemistry, function, and clinical relevance. Bone 1998;22:181–187.

20 Light ND, Bailey AJ: The chemistry of the collagen cross-links. Purification and characterization of cross-linked polymeric peptide material from mature collagen containing unknown amino acids. Biochem J 1980;185:373–381.
21 Reiser K, McCormick RJ, Rucker RB: Enzymatic and nonenzymatic cross-linking of collagen and elastin. FASEB J 1992;6:2439–2449.
22 Saito M, Marumo K: Collagen cross-links as a determinant of bone quality: a possible explanation for bone fragility in aging, osteoporosis, and diabetes mellitus. Osteoporos Int 2010;21:195–214.
23 Panwar P, Du X, Sharma V, Lamour G, Castro M, Li H, et al: Effects of cysteine proteases on the structural and mechanical properties of collagen fibers. J Biol Chem 2013;288:5940–5950.
24 Torzilli PA, Arduino JM, Gregory JD, Bansal M: Effect of proteoglycan removal on solute mobility in articular cartilage. J Biomech 1997;30:895–902.
25 Suppa P, Ruggeri A Jr, Tay FR, Prati C, Biasotto M, Falconi M, et al: Reduced antigenicity of type I collagen and proteoglycans in sclerotic dentin. J Dent Res 2006;85:133–137.
26 Dimuzio MT, Veis A: Phosphophoryns-major noncollagenous proteins of rat incisor dentin. Calcif Tissue Res 1978; 25:169–178.
27 Gusman H, Santana RB, Zehnder M: Matrix metalloproteinase levels and gelatinolytic activity in clinically healthy and inflamed human dental pulps. Eur J Oral Sci 2002;110:353–357.
28 Sorsa T, Tjaderhane L, Salo T: Matrix metalloproteinases (MMPs) in oral diseases. Oral Dis 2004;10:311–318.
29 Martin-De Las Heras S, Valenzuela A, Overall CM: The matrix metalloproteinase gelatinase A in human dentine. Arch Oral Biol 2000;45:757–765.
30 Mazzoni A, Papa V, Nato F, Carrilho M, Tjäderhane L, Ruggeri A Jr, et al: Immunohistochemical and biochemical assay of MMP-3 in human dentine. J Dent 2011;39:231–237.
31 Sulkala M, Tervahartiala T, Sorsa T, Larmas M, Salo T, Tjaderhane L: Matrix metalloproteinase-8 (MMP-8) is the major collagenase in human dentin. Arch Oral Biol 2007;52:121–127.
32 Nascimento FD, Minciotti CL, Geraldeli S, Carrilho MR, Pashley DH, Tay FR, et al: Cysteine cathepsins in human carious dentin. J Dent Res 2011;90:506–511.
33 Tersariol IL, Geraldeli S, Minciotti CL, Nascimento FD, Paakkonen V, Martins MT, et al: Cysteine cathepsins in human dentin-pulp complex. J Endod 2010;36: 475–481.
34 Bedran-Russo AK, Pauli GF, Chen SN, McAlpine J, Castellan CS, Phansalkar RS, et al: Dentin biomodification: strategies, renewable resources and clinical applications. Dent Mater 2014;30:62–76.
35 Foote CS: Mechanisms of photosensitized oxidation. There are several different types of photosensitized oxidation which may be important in biological systems. Science 1968;162:963–970.
36 Barnard K, Light ND, Sims TJ, Bailey AJ: Chemistry of the collagen cross-links. Origin and partial characterization of a putative mature cross-link of collagen. Biochem J 1987;244:303–309.
37 Snibson GR: Collagen cross-linking: a new treatment paradigm in corneal disease – a review. Clin Exp Ophthalmol 2010;38:141–153.
38 McCall AS, Kraft S, Edelhauser HF, Kidder GW, Lundquist RR, Bradshaw HE, et al: Mechanisms of corneal tissue cross-linking in response to treatment with topical riboflavin and long-wavelength ultraviolet radiation (UVA). Invest Ophthalmol Vis Sci 2010;51:129–138.
39 Fawzy A, Nitisusanta L, Iqbal K, Daood U, Beng LT, Neo J: Characterization of riboflavin-modified dentin collagen matrix. J Dent Res 2012;91:1049–1054.
40 Cheung DT, Perelman N, Ko EC, Nimni ME: Mechanism of crosslinking of proteins by glutaraldehyde III. Reaction with collagen in tissues. Connect Tissue Res 1985;13:109–115.
41 Cheung DT, Tong D, Perelman N, Ertl D, Nimni ME: Mechanism of crosslinking of proteins by glutaraldehyde. IV: In vitro and in vivo stability of a cross-linked collagen matrix. Connect Tissue Res 1990;25:27–34.
42 Bedran-Russo AK, Pashley DH, Agee K, Drummond JL, Miescke KJ: Changes in stiffness of demineralized dentin following application of collagen crosslinkers. J Biomed Mater Res B Appl Biomater 2008;86:330–334.
43 Han B, Jaurequi J, Tang BW, Nimni ME: Proanthocyanidin: a natural crosslinking reagent for stabilizing collagen matrices. J Biomed Mater Res A 2003;65: 118–124.
44 Olde Damink LH, Dijkstra PJ, van Luyn MJ, van Wachem PB, Nieuwenhuis P, Feijen J: Cross-linking of dermal sheep collagen using a water-soluble carbodiimide. Biomaterials 1996;17:765–773.
45 Staros JV, Wright RW, Swingle DM: Enhancement by N-hydroxysulfosuccinimide of water-soluble carbodiimide-mediated coupling reactions. Anal Biochem 1986;156:220–222.
46 Bedran-Russo AK, Vidal CM, Dos Santos PH, Castellan CS: Long-term effect of carbodiimide on dentin matrix and resin-dentin bonds. J Biomed Mater Res B Appl Biomater 2010;94:250–255.
47 Petite H, Duval JL, Frei V, Abdul-Malak N, Sigot-Luizard MF, Herbage D: Cytocompatibility of calf pericardium treated by glutaraldehyde and by the acyl azide methods in an organotypic culture model. Biomaterials 1995;16:1003–1008.
48 Scheffel DL, Hebling J, Scheffel RH, Agee K, Turco G, de Souza Costa CA, et al: Inactivation of matrix-bound matrix metalloproteinases by cross-linking agents in acid-etched dentin. Oper Dent 2014;39:152–158.
49 Trouet AU, Pirson P, Steiger R, Masquelier M, Baurain R, Gillet J: Development of new derivatives of primaquine by association with lysosomotropic carriers. Bull World Health Organ 1981;59:449–458.
50 Sung HW, Chang WH, Ma CY, Lee MH: Crosslinking of biological tissues using genipin and/or carbodiimide. J Biomed Mater Res A 2003;64:427–438.
51 Sung HW, Chang Y, Chiu CT, Chen CN, Liang HC: Crosslinking characteristics and mechanical properties of a bovine pericardium fixed with a naturally occurring crosslinking agent. J Biomed Mater Res 1999;47:116–126.
52 Pandey KB, Rizvi SI: Plant polyphenols as dietary antioxidants in human health and disease. Oxid Med Cell Longev 2009;2:270–278.
53 Ferreira D, Slade D, Marais JPJ: Flavans and proanthocyanidins; in Anderson OM, Markham KR (eds): The Flavonoids–Chemistry, Biochemistry and Applications. Boca Raton, FL, CRC Taylor & Francis, 2006, pp 553–616.
54 Cao N, Fu Y, He J: Mechanical properties of gelatin films cross-linked, respectively, by ferulic acid and tannin acid. Food Hydrocolloids 2007;21:575–584.
55 Hagerman AE, Klucher KM: Tannin-protein interactions. Prog Clin Biol Res 1986;213:67–76.

56 Vidal CM, Zhu W, Manohar S, Aydin B, Keiderling TA, Messersmith PB, et al: Collagen-collagen interactions mediated by plant-derived proanthocyanidins: a spectroscopic and atomic force microscopy study. Acta Biomater 2016;41:110–118.
57 Hagerman AE, Butler LG: The specificity of proanthocyanidin-protein interactions. J Biol Chem 1981;256:4494–4497.
58 Bedran-Russo AK, Castellan CS, Shinohara MS, Hassan L, Antunes A: Characterization of biomodified dentin matrices for potential preventive and reparative therapies. Acta Biomater 2011;7:1735–1741.
59 Epasinghe DJ, Yiu CK, Burrow MF, Hiraishi N, Tay FR: The inhibitory effect of proanthocyanidin on soluble and collagen-bound proteases. J Dent 2013;41: 832–839.
60 Vidal CM, Aguiar TR, Phansalkar R, McAlpine JB, Napolitano JG, Chen SN, et al: Galloyl moieties enhance the dentin biomodification potential of plant-derived catechins. Acta Biomater 2014; 10:3288–3294.
61 Macedo GV, Yamauchi M, Bedran-Russo AK: Effects of chemical cross-linkers on caries-affected dentin bonding. J Dent Res 2009;88:1096–1100.
62 Leme-Kraus AA, Aydin B, Vidal CM, Phansalkar RM, Nam JW, McAlpine J, et al: Biostability of the proanthocyanidins-dentin complex and adhesion studies. J Dent Res 2016;96:406–412.
63 Walter R, Miguez PA, Arnold RR, Pereira PN, Duarte WR, Yamauchi M: Effects of natural cross-linkers on the stability of dentin collagen and the inhibition of root caries in vitro. Caries Res 2008;42:263–268.
64 Kim GE, Leme-Kraus AA, Phansalkar R, Viana G, Wu C, Chen SN, et al: Effect of bioactive primers on bacterial-induced secondary caries at the tooth-resin interface. Oper Dent 2017;42:196–202.
65 Xie Q, Bedran-Russo AK, Wu CD: In vitro remineralization effects of grape seed extract on artificial root caries. J Dent 2008;36:900–906.
66 Pavan S, Xie Q, Hara AT, Bedran-Russo AK: Biomimetic approach for root caries prevention using a proanthocyanidin-rich agent. Caries Res 2011;45:443–447.
67 Hiraishi N, Sono R, Islam MS, Otsuki M, Tagami J, Takatsuka T: Effect of hesperidin in vitro on root dentine collagen and demineralization. J Dent 2011;39:391–396.
68 Epasinghe DJ, Yiu C, Burrow MF: Effect of flavonoids on remineralization of artificial root caries. Aust Dent J 2016; 61:196–202.
69 Epasinghe DJ, Kwan S, Chu D, Lei MM, Burrow MF, Yiu CK: Synergistic effects of proanthocyanidin, tri-calcium phosphate and fluoride on artificial root caries and dentine collagen. Mater Sci Eng C Mater Biol Appl 2017;73:293–299.

Ana K. Bedran-Russo, DDS, MS, PhD
Department of Restorative Dentistry, University of Illinois at Chicago
801 S. Paulina Street, Room 531a
Chicago, IL 60612 (USA)
E-Mail bedran@uic.edu

Carrilho MRO (ed): Root Caries: From Prevalence to Therapy.
Monogr Oral Sci. Basel, Karger, 2017, vol 26, pp 106–114 (DOI: 10.1159/000479352)

Management of Cavitated Root Caries Lesions: Minimum Intervention and Alternatives

Michael F. Burrow[a, b] · Margaret A. Stacey[a]

[a]Melbourne Dental School, The University of Melbourne, Melbourne, VIC, Australia; [b]Faculty of Dentistry, University of Hong Kong, Hong Kong, China

Abstract

The prevalence of root caries among the elderly is increasing. The lesion shape can vary considerably from a broad shallow saucer-shape to a deeper defined cavity. The variety of shapes poses a series of complications when considering restorative management. This is accompanied with a paucity of clinical evidence on treatment techniques and clinical outcomes. The current philosophy centered on conservative management of root caries will most likely provide patients with the greatest chance of maintaining their teeth. When a lesion can be effectively cleaned in conjunction with a high fluoride content toothpaste and other remineralizing agents, this should be the treatment of choice. For lesions that are cavitated and cannot be effectively cleaned, the initial management should be to apply remineralizing agents for a period to "harden" lesion margins thus potentially reducing the prepared cavity and restoration size, as well as providing a better-defined tooth-restoration margin for finishing. Material selection is either a glass ionomer cement (conventional or resin-modified) or resin-based material. Frequently, the restoration site is easily contaminated; hence, glass ionomer cement is an ideal material. However, for saliva-deficient patients, resin composite or a combination of resin composite and resin-modified glass ionomer adhesive allows for a highly polished, easily cleansable restoration surface that may reduce the potential for further caries initiation. The current evidence base for the restoration of root caries is poor.

Introduction

As the population is aging worldwide, the associated advances in the management of dental diseases have led to many people retaining their teeth for life; thus, the prevalence of root caries has been increasing [1–3]. The current evidence indicates that patients with a prior history of coronal caries, poor plaque control, and dry mouth also show an increased risk of developing root caries [3]. However, there are patients with exposed root surfaces owing to periodontal attachment loss who present with root caries requiring some form of intervention even though they have experienced minimal coronal caries. In addition, as the number of patients retaining most of their teeth increases, there is also an associated increase in the exposed root surfaces that may be susceptible to caries [4].

The primary aim of the treatment should be centered on Minimal Treatment, as originally coined by Mount [5] or "Minimal Intervention Dentistry (MID)" which was described by Dawson and Makinson [6, 7] in the early 90's. This chapter focuses on the minimal operative interventions and aspects of MID in relation to the management of cavitated root caries lesions.

One of the major difficulties with managing the root caries lesion is its lateral spread rather than lesion depth. In association with this, a laboratory-based study investigating artificial root lesion formation showed that lesion depth was significantly greater in the absence of cementum [8]. Therefore, patients who have undergone extensive periodontal therapy may fall into this group and possibly be at greater risk. Typically, root caries lesions are broad and shallow, often leading to encirclement or 'ring barking' of curved root surfaces (Fig. 1).

For the purposes of this chapter, it is important to understand what is meant by a "cavitated root caries lesion." Cavitated lesions typically take 2 presentations. As noted in Figure 1, many lesions are shallow and saucer-shaped, extending around a large part of the root surface. The curvature of the root and frequently indistinct lesion borders make restoration placement and finishing difficult. Often these lesions can be easily cleansed of the biofilm if accessible to a toothbrush. However, occasionally these lesions may also have a deeper portion that cannot be easily cleansed, this is the second presentation form, namely a distinct cavity. These deeper lesions are often located on approximal surfaces of molars just below the gingival margin where a toothbrush is unable to access the lesion, particularly the deepest parts. Visual and tactile detections are often difficult, and the cavitated lesions may be found only after viewing a bitewing radiograph. They appear well defined, are located a long way gingivally from the marginal ridge of the tooth. Such lesions have a high probability of pulp exposure and usually need to be restored as soon as they are identified (Fig. 2).

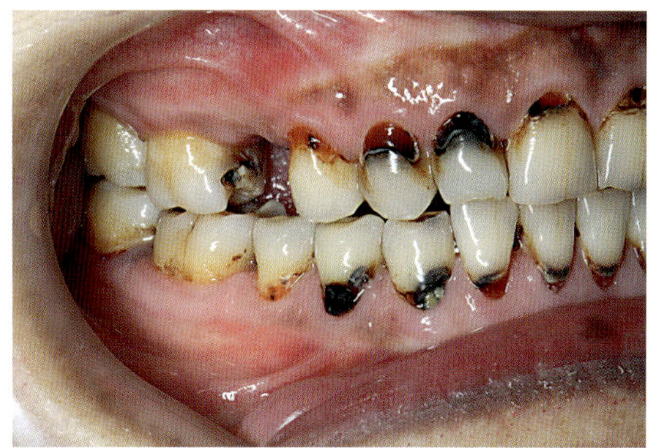

Fig. 1. Note the extent of the caries lesions around the circumference of the teeth caused by the consumption of cola drinks. The shape extends around the curved tooth surface making restoration difficult.

Cavitated Lesion Management

A variety of methods can be used for the management of cavitated lesions. The principal ethos of management must be centered on minimal intervention techniques aimed at maximum conservation of tooth tissue, that is, where possible surgical management of the lesion should be a last resort. Frequently, a combination of initial remineralization followed by surgical intervention should occur to minimize the size of the cavity and for restoration.

Biofilm Disruption

Cavitated lesions, even up to the depth of approximately 2 mm, should be assessed to determine if a toothbrush can reliably remove the biofilm on the whole lesion surface. If biofilm removal can be

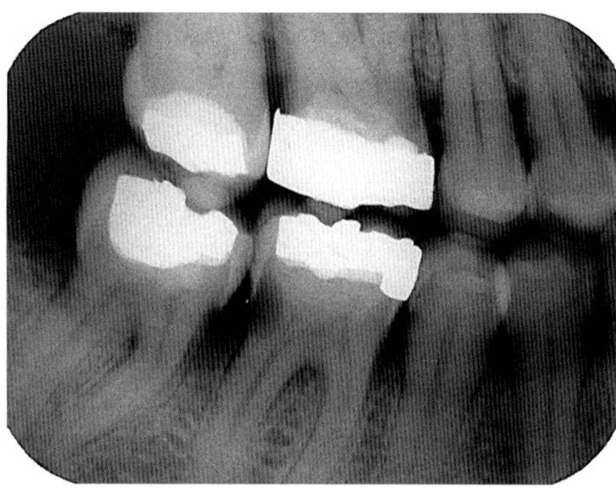

Fig. 2. Tooth 46, note the extent of the well-defined lesion on the distal surface. Also distal of 45, 14, and 15 have early lesions that need to be checked clinically. Due to the depth from the occlusal surface (marginal ridge) and subgingival position, restoration of these lesions is difficult. Intervention can be destructive of tooth structure and pulp exposure is highly likely.

consistently achieved by a patient, then this non-invasive method is potentially the best form of lesion management. Regular biofilm removal with a high fluoride content toothpaste, for example, 5,000 ppm, and use of other remineralizing agents such as Ca and PO_4 containing crèmes should be instituted [9, 10]. In addition, toothbrushing abrades the softened lesion surface exposing the underlying harder higher mineral content tooth tissue. The only negative impact is the lesion will frequently darken in color over time as the mineral content on the surface of the lesion increases and possibly extrinsic stains are incorporated into the arresting lesion. This method can be one of the most effective ways of managing these lesions and avoiding the need for a restoration. If aesthetics becomes an issue for the patient, then a minimal tooth-colored restoration may be placed.

"Lesion Exposure" Method

In some cases, where lesions have shallow cavitation but extend beneath the enamel, rather than excavating the carious tissue, a minimal surgical approach can be used that exposes the dentin lesion by removing only the overlying unsupported enamel. The process is undertaken without the need for local analgesia by using a fine-grit tapered or flame-shaped diamond bur under air-water spray in either a low or intermediate (1:5 increase) speed hand piece. After exposure of the dentin lesion, the patient is given lesion-specific oral hygiene instruction using high fluoride toothpastes. Over time, the action of the toothbrush will abrade the softened surface exposing the underlying harder dentin which remineralizes. The lesion gradually darkens and becomes arrested if the patient complies with and can effectively implement the lesion-specific hygiene regimen. It would also be feasible to treat the exposed dentin lesion with a silver diamine fluoride (SDF) solution, however, the resulting compromised aesthetics must be taken into consideration. The additional use of Ca and PO_4 containing crèmes can also aid in remineralizing these lesions. Figure 3 shows a case of a patient 10 years post-radiation therapy, where the "lesion exposure" method was used. It can be seen how the dentin lesion is exposed to the oral cavity, then careful biofilm removal using a 5,000 ppm toothpaste in association with the CPP-ACP containing remineralizing agent (Tooth Mousse, GC Corp, Japan) has led to the lesions arresting and slowly increasing in surface hardness. The method is simple, involves minimal destruction of tooth tissue, and rarely necessitates the placement of a restoration.

Caries Excavation and Restoration

When excavating the dentin, the aim should be to avoid pulp exposure. A recent study investigating deep coronal lesions in molar teeth showed that in a percentage of cases, even teeth exhibiting periapical lesions on cone beam computed tomography images, were able to be "healed" as determined by the disappearance of the periapical lesions, after using either a refined calcium

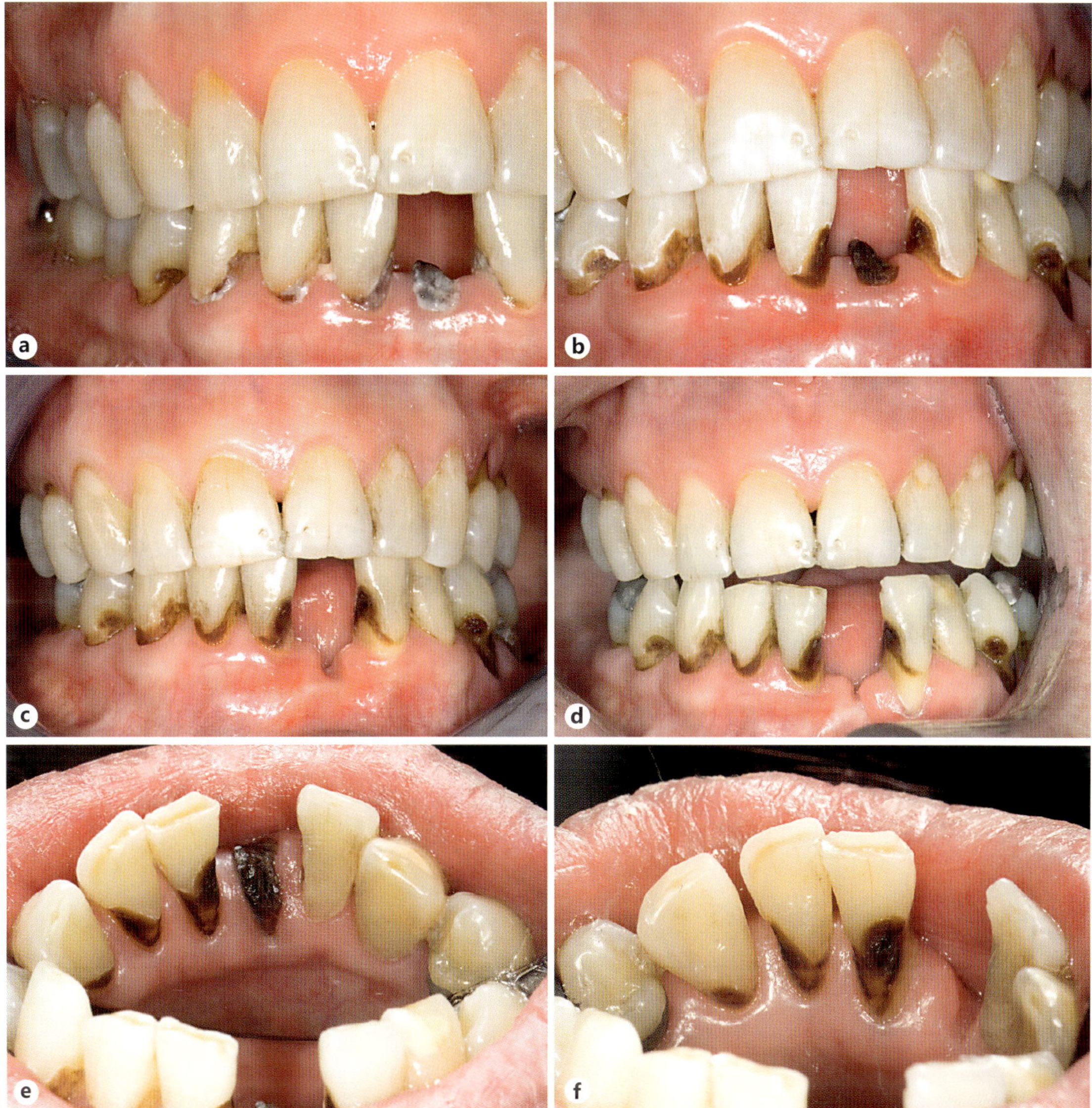

Fig. 3. a Labial view, before lesion exposure; (**b**) labial view, after lesion exposure. The enamel was trimmed using a slow-speed fine-grit diamond to expose the underlying carious tissue; (**c**) labial view, 4 months after lesion exposure; (**d**) labial view 7 months after lesion exposure. The toothbrush has abraded the soft surface, exposing the carious dentin which has become darker, smoother, and harder; (**e**) lingual view, after lesion exposure; (**f**) lingual view, 4 months after lesion exposure.

silicate cement (Biodentine, Septodont, Saint Maur des Fosses, France) or conventional glass ionomer cement (GIC) (Fuji XI GP, GC Corp, Tokyo, Japan) [11]. It is possible that this same method could be applicable for the management of deeper root lesions. However, one clinical evaluation comparing GIC with Biodentine on root caries lesions showed that the GIC was much more effective from the aspect of restoration survival [12].

The concept of preserving dentin that may still contain bacteria in a cavity beneath a sealed restoration should be the aim of managing these deeper lesions. However, material selection to restore such a dentin cavity is important. This dentin has a reduced mineral content and an increased moisture content; thus, resin-based adhesive restorative materials are not the ideal option. These lesions should be restored with a GIC (conventional or resin-modified) or possibly a refined calcium silicate cement. However, a much better clinical evidence base is needed.

Caries excavation and cavity preparation will be dependent on the location of the lesion. Typically, lesions located on the labial/buccal surface of a tooth can be managed conservatively by excavating only the deeper, non-cleansable portion of the lesion. The carious tissue may be excavated with either slow-speed (round) burs or hand instruments.

For posterior approximal root surface lesions, management is often more complex. Careful assessment should be made at the examination stage. If the lesion can be identified visually from the buccal or lingual embrasure, then caries excavation could be undertaken from the embrasure. Otherwise, it may be necessary to access the lesion from the occlusal surface through the marginal ridge. This method is often very destructive of tooth tissue, and the restoration is often not well supported at the gingival margin as the gingival floor is typically quite narrow. Matrix positioning and placement is frequently difficult, which in turn makes material insertion into the deep narrow cavity difficult. Often a 2-stage placement of the restorative material is needed. This method fills no more than the lower third in height of the cavity with the selected restorative material and allows it to set. The matrix band is loosened, moved occlusally and stabilized, then the remainder of the cavity is restored and contoured. This technique makes it easier to attain a well-contoured, easily cleansable, proximal surface; it also ensures that a tight contact area is achieved.

Chemomechanical Caries Excavation

Although the use of chemomechanical caries excavation has not been widely accepted by the profession, it is a useful and simple option. Two broad types of solution are available. The first is the sodium hypochlorite-based material, Carisolv (MediTeam Dental AB, Sweden). Carisolv has been available for many years and there have been several iterations of its formulation. The second is the enzyme-based solution, Papacarie (Fórmula and Ação, Brazil). This more recent material uses enzymes from the leaves of the Papaya tree. Recent research has shown both of these materials can be effective in removing the denatured carious dentin, often leaving a thicker layer of the mineral depleted carious dentin compared with rotary instrument excavation [13]. The chemomechanical method can, therefore, provide a more conservative cavity preparation with a reduced chance of pulp exposure. This method does not require specialized equipment, such as hand pieces. Both are gels that allow easy placement into a cavity and removal of the dentin with hand instruments without the need for local analgesia. Such a method is ideal for managing caries in patients who may not be able to attend a dental office for treatment, for example, home-bound special needs patients or the elderly.

Atraumatic Restorative Technique

The atraumatic restorative technique (ART) philosophy grew at about the same time MID also became popular. The method was essentially aimed at providing a simple means of caries management, where dental facilities were limited or non-existent. The method of simply removing unsupported enamel and the softened carious tissue with hand instruments followed by restoration has shown excellent outcomes for the management of coronal carious lesions [14]. However, most studies have concentrated on the management of occlusal caries in young populations. More recently, studies have looked at ART for the elderly and provided encouraging results [15–17]. The ART method has also been adopted with the use of a chemomechanical caries method in a study for the management of root caries lesions in the elderly. This study compared the standard ART method of hand excavation of the soft caries with ART using a chemochemical method of caries excavation with Carisolv [18]. This 2-year study showed an overall 63% survival rate of restorations. The same degree of restoration survival was achieved when Carisolv was used. The ART method is promising as a means of management of cavitated root caries lesions and may be a useful alternative for institutionalized patients unable to attend a dental office.

Material Selection

The advent of adhesive dental materials has made the use (placement) and choice of materials simpler for restoration of root caries lesions. Before these materials were available, the only material available was silver amalgam. Silver amalgam has some useful properties in that the corrosion products probably help reduce the recurrence of caries around restoration margins as well as affect the growth of the biofilm [19]. The one great disadvantage is its non-adhesive nature. Cavities must have a well-defined retention form and be deep enough to give the amalgam strength even though the restoration is usually not load bearing. Cavity preparation for amalgam requires the removal of sound tooth structure as well as marginal extension to sound tooth structure, which is difficult for root lesions due to the shallow ill-defined borders of the lesions. However, the adhesive restorative materials can be placed in quite thin layers and can avoid the loss of tissue that can be easily remineralized.

The 2 most commonly used options are now GIC, either the conventional or resin-modified versions, or resin-based materials with the use of an enamel/dentin bonding agent. Unfortunately, scant evidence evaluating the clinical use of these materials for the management of root caries exists. Almost all studies on root dentin have used non-carious cervical lesions that are comprised of sclerotic dentin. These studies cannot be extrapolated, as the dentin substrate is very different from root caries, which is mineral depleted dentin, the opposite of the non-carious cervical lesion, which is typically highly mineralized. Studies of posterior resin composite restorations usually have enamel margins, so these too cannot be extrapolated to root restorations where the cavo-surface margin is on cementum or dentin.

Therefore, when restoring a root lesion, the gingival margin position, probability of moisture contamination, and potential for gingival bleeding must be considered. Where moisture control is difficult to manage, the use of a resin-based system is contraindicated. This only leaves the option of GIC. The dentin surface should be conditioned with polyacrylic acid (PAA) as a means to prepare the dentin to bond to the GIC as PAA starts to interact with the calcium in the tooth mineral via an ionic interaction, thus aiding better adhesion [20]. PAA conditioning also helps clean the cavity and remove any blood or saliva contamination that may inhibit adhesion on the dentin. The choice of resin-modified or conventional GIC is often related to a personal preference, whether a light-curing unit is available, and the depth of the cavity. Cavity depth is critical for the light-cured resin-modified GICs as attenuation of the light intensity may lead to the resin component not curing to its fullest extent for deep posterior root lesions. The current fast-setting conventional GICs that exhibit good strength and higher fluoride release are the material of choice for patients with normal saliva flow, or where the gingival floor of an approximal cavity extends greater than 4.5 mm below the occlusal surface of the tooth. An adjunct treatment to possibly reduce caries formation around the margins of these restorations can be the application of SDF to the cavity walls prior to restoration placement. A recent laboratory study comparing the progression of artificial dentin caries lesions restored with either a CPP-ACP containing or conventional glass ionomer cement, with and without the application of 38% SDF to the cavity walls prior to GIC placement showed that both SDF treatment and incorporation of CPP-ACP into the GIC restorative material were able to slow deterioration and demineralization around the restoration margins [21]. Furthermore laboratory data show that the adhesion of tooth-colored materials is not compromised by SDF application to non-carious dentin [22]. The use of SDF on cavity walls has yet to be evaluated clinically, but the laboratory-based results show promise and may also be an option for lesions requiring restoration in patients whose oral hygiene effectiveness or compliance may be compromised. However, for those patients where saliva flow is compromised (determined after appropriate testing), it seems that GICs may not be the best option due to their susceptibility to surface dissolution. One means of slowing the dissolution is to coat the GIC with a proprietary resin-coating, for example, G-Coat Plus (GC Corp, Japan). This has been shown to protect the surface from wear, as well as provide a slightly smoother surface that will make biofilm removal easier and reduce the effects of localized acid attack (Fig. 4).

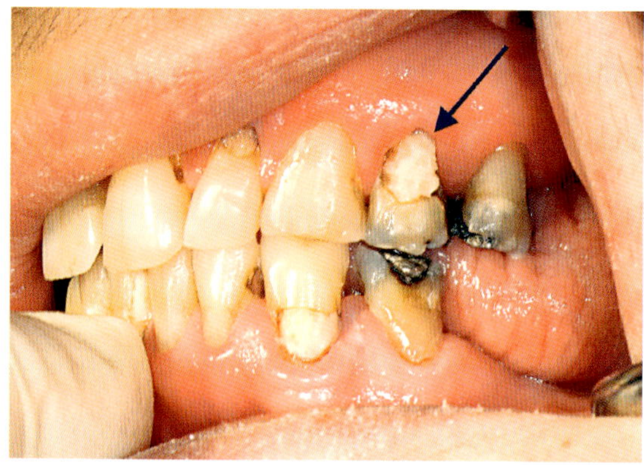

Fig. 4. Glass ionomer cement restorations may be eroded rapidly when the saliva flow is compromised, as demonstrated by the conventional GIC restoration in tooth 24 inserted 33 months prior to this photograph. (Arrow) Placing a resin coating will assist in reducing the rate of dissolution, but fluoride release will also be reduced.

For resin-based materials, it must be remembered that the cavity margin is likely to be demineralized dentin, possibly with some poor-quality enamel at the occlusal margin. Ideally, remineralizing treatments should be used to "harden" the surrounding demineralized tissues for a period prior to cavity preparation and restoration. Excellent moisture control is essential to achieve reliable bonding. The option of an etch-and-rinse or self-etch system needs to be considered. Current evidence suggests that a 3-step etch and rinse system will provide the best results [23]. For the self-etch option, a 2-step self-etch system is ideal. Again, the evidence is limited, with studies on restoring this part of the tooth centered on non-carious cervical lesions.

Choice of the type of composite restorative material, flowable versus microfill versus nano- or microhybrid, remains controversial. The most important consideration for composite selection is whether the material is able to be polished to a very high polish with smooth margins. This will facilitate biofilm removal by the patient, thereby reducing the chances of new demineralization occurring at restoration margins. While the use of composites will provide the best aesthetic option, the evidence remains limited as to whether a fluoride-releasing composite will provide any inhibition of marginal demineralization [24].

A third option exists where a resin-modified glass ionomer adhesive, for example, Fuji Bond LC (GC Corp), or Riva Bond LC, (SDI Pty Ltd, Bayswater, Australia) can be used to bond to the root dentin and the cavity then filled with a resin composite. This provides the clinician with the advantages of reliable bonding to the root dentin via the GIC, maximum aesthetics, and a smooth margin with the resin composite. Two studies have shown good restoration survival when placed in NCCLs for 5 and 6 years. Hence, this method may be good for root caries patients with salivary deficiency [25, 26].

For the deep posterior approximal root caries cavity, depth of cure must again be considered. There is now a resin-modified auto (self)-cured GIC available that can be used instead of a light-cured resin-modified GIC. This can be used with the laminate (sandwich) technique, where the GIC is placed in the bottom third of the cavity, then a resin adhesive and composite filling is placed in the occlusal two-thirds. It is important, however, to monitor these restorations to ensure that surface dissolution of the GIC is not occurring [27]. When surface dissolution is identified, then a repair to the restoration should be undertaken.

Conclusion

A variety of options exist for the restorative management of root caries lesions. Where the lesion is shallow and broad, the most conservative option of remineralization and arresting the lesion is the option of choice. Lesions that undermine enamel can be managed by the judicious removal of unsupported enamel followed by the non-surgical management to arrest lesion activity. For deeper non-cleansable lesions, initial remineralization of margins should be attempted followed by placement of a smaller tooth-colored restoration. Frequently the material of choice is a GIC, but for saliva-deficient patients a highly-polished resin composite bonded with either an enamel/dentin adhesive or resin-modified GIC adhesive seems to the optimum material. However, evidence on restoration survival and caries risk is still lacking.

References

1 Silva M, Hopcraft M, Morgan M: Dental Caries in Victorian nursing homes. Aust Dent J 2014;59:321–328.

2 Amer RS, Kolker JL: Restoration of root surface caries in vulnerable elderly patients: a review of the literature. Spec Care Dentist 2013;33:141–149.

3 Hayes M, Da Mata C, Cole M, McKenna G, Burke F, Allen PF: Risk indicators associated with root caries in independently living older adults. J Dent 2015; 51:8–14.

4 McNally ME, Matthews DC, Clovis JB, Brillant M, Filiaggi MJ: The oral health of ageing baby boomers: a comparison of adults aged 45–64 and those 65 years and older. Gerodontol 2014;31:123–135.

5 Mount GJ: Minimal treatment of the carious lesion. Int Dent J 1991;41:55–59.

6 Dawson AS, Makinson OF: Dental treatment and dental health. Part 1. A review of studies in support of a philosophy of Minimum Intervention Dentistry. Aust Dent J 1992;37:126–132.

7 Dawson AS, Makinson OF: Dental treatment and dental health. Part 2. An alternative philosophy and some new treatment modalities in operative dentistry. Aust Dent J 1992;37:205–210.

8 Smith PW, Preston KP, Higham SM: Development of an in situ root caries model. A. In vitro investigations. J Dent 2005;33:253–267.

9 Ekstrand KR, Ekstrand ML, Lykkeaa J, Bardow A, Twetman S: Whole-saliva fluoride levels and saturation indices in 65+ elderly during use of four different toothpaste regimens. Caries Res 2015; 49:489–498.

10 Ekstrand KR: High fluoride dentifrices for elderly and vulnerable adults: does it work and if so, then why? Care Res 2016;50(suppl 1):15–21.

11 Hashem D, Mannocci F, Patel S, Manoharan A, Brown JE, Watson TF, Banerjee A: Clinical and radiographic assessment of the efficacy of calcium silicate indirect pulp capping: a randomized controlled clinical trial. J Dent Res 2015; 94:562–568.

12 Hayes M, da Mata C, Tada S, Cole M, McKenna G, Burke FM, Allen PF: Evaluation of Biodentine in the restoration of root caries: a randomized controlled trial. J Dent Res Clin Trans Res 2016;1: 51–58.

13 Hamama HH, Yiu CK, Burrow MF, King NM: Chemical, morphological and microhardness changes of dentine after chemomechanical caries removal. Aust Dent J 2013;58:283–292.

14 Frencken JE, Leal SC, Navarro MF: Twenty-five-year atraumatic restorative treatment (ART) approach: a comprehensive overview. Clin Oral Investig 2012;16:1337–1346.

15 da Mata C, Allen PF, Cronin M, O'Mahony D, McKenna G, Woods N: Cost-effectiveness of ART restorations in elderly adults: a randomized clinical trial. Community Dent Oral Epidemiol 2014;42:79–87.

16 da Mata C, Allen PF, Cronin M, O'Mahony D, McKenna G, Woods N: Two-year survival of ART restorations placed in elderly patients: a randomised controlled clinical trial. J Dent 2015;43: 405–411.

17 Cruz Gonzalez AC, Marin Zuluaga DJ: Clinical outcome of root caries restorations using ART and rotary techniques in institutionalized elders. Braz Oral Res 2016;30:pii: S1806-83242016000100260.
18 Gil-Montoya JA, Mateos-Palacios R, Bravo M, Gonzalez-Mole MA, Pulgar R: Atraumatic restorative treatment and Carisolv use for root caries in the elderly: 2-year follow-up randomized clinical trial. Clin Oral Investig 2014;18:1089–1095.
19 Beyth N, Domb AJ, Weiss EI: An in vitro quantitative antibacterial analysis of amalgam and composite resins. J Dent 2007;35:201–206.
20 Es-Souni M, Fischer-Brandies H, Zaporojshenko V, Es-Souni M: On the interaction of polyacrylic acid as a conditioning agent with bovine enamel. Biomaterials 2002;23:2871–2878.
21 Zhao IS, Mei ML, Burrow MF, Lo EC, Chu CH: Prevention of secondary caries using silver diamine fluoride treatment and casein phosphopeptide-amorphous calcium phosphate modified glass-ionomer cement. J Dent 2017;57:38–44.
22 Quock RL, Barros JA, Yang SW, Patel SA: Effect of silver diamine fluoride on microtensile bond strength to dentin. Oper Dent 2012;37:610–616.
23 Peumans M, De Munck J, Mine A, Van Meerbeek B: Clinical effectiveness of contemporary adhesives for the restoration of non-carious cervical lesions. A systematic review. Dent Mater 2014;30: 1089–1103.
24 Cury JA, de Oliveira BH, dos Santos AP, Tenuta LM: Are fluoride releasing dental materials clinically effective on caries control? Dent Mater 2016;32:323–333.
25 Tyas MJ, Burrow MF: Clinical evaluation of a resin-modified glass ionomer adhesive system: results at five years. Oper Dent 2002;27:438–441.
26 van Dijken JW: Retention of a resin-modified glass ionomer adhesive in non-carious cervical lesions. A 6-year follow-up. J Dent 2005;33:541–547.
27 Kirsten GA, Rached RN, Mazur RF, Vieira S, Souza EM: Effect of open-sandwich vs. adhesive restorative techniques on enamel and dentine demineralization: an in situ study. J Dent 2013;41: 872–880.

Michael Francis Burrow
Faculty of Dentistry, The University of Hong Kong
Prince Philip Dental Hospital
34 Hospital Road
Sai Ying Pun, Hong Kong (China)
E-Mail mfburr58@hku.hk

Carrilho MRO (ed): Root Caries: From Prevalence to Therapy.
Monogr Oral Sci. Basel, Karger, 2017, vol 26, pp 115–124 (DOI: 10.1159/000479353)

Clinical Performance of Root Surface Restorations

Alessandra Reis[a] • Paulo Vinícius Soares[c] • Juliana de Geus[b] • Alessandro D. Loguercio[a]

[a]Department of Restorative Dentistry, State University of Ponta Grossa, Ponta Grossa, and [b]Paulo Picanço Faculty, Fortaleza, and [c]Professor at Operative Dentistry and Dental Materials Department, Coordinator of NCCL Research Group, School of Dentistry, Federal University of Uberlândia, Uberlândia, Brazil

Abstract

This chapter describes the clinical performance of restorations placed in root caries lesions. The prevalence of root caries and other types of cervical lesions, caused by abfraction, erosion, and abrasion (non-carious cervical lesions) are high, mainly in the elderly; and therefore, restorative procedures are indicated. We will revise the restorative materials used to restore these types of lesions and present evidence-based findings to provide clinicians with better evidence for choosing them. Additionally, some steps of the restorative procedure for the placement of resin-based composites will be revised and common clinical questions related to these steps will be answered based on high evidence level, produced by randomized clinical trials and systematic reviews of the literature.

Introduction

Root caries lesions and non-carious cervical lesions (NCCLs) are prevalent diseases that affect the cervical and root areas of the teeth (Fig. 1–3). In many cases, they occur simultaneously (Fig. 1). For instance, a recent study [1] reported that the prevalence of root caries in elderly individuals aged 60 years and above, residing in Bangalore city (India) was 46.4%. In the rural health center in India, the prevalence of root caries was 41.9% [2]. In Japan, about 39% of the subjects had one or more decayed roots [3]. A higher prevalence was reported in Sri Lanka, with root surface caries of 89.7% in subjects aged 60 years and above. In a Brazilian sample of 50–59 years, a total of 78.1% had at least one root caries lesion [4].

When it comes to NCCLs, these figures are also high. In middle-aged and elderly populations of China, the prevalence of NCCLs was 76.8 and 81.3%, respectively [5]. In another study in China, clinical assessment showed that the overall prevalence of subjects diagnosed with NCCLs was 63%, regardless of age. However, other studies point out that these lesions are more prevalent in elderly patients [5]. Only 22.7% of adolescents ranging from 12 to 15 years old presented NCCLs [6].

Several risk factors such as age, location (more common in first premolars, canines, and second premolars), frequency of toothbrushing, bruxism, and family income were found to be associated with NCCLs [7]. In regard to root carious, tobacco use and alcohol consumption, as well as wearing dentures, were significantly associated

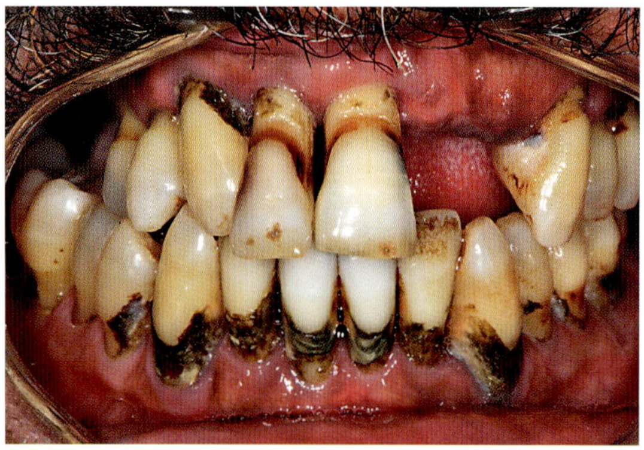

Fig. 1. Root caries associated with non-carious cervical lesions.

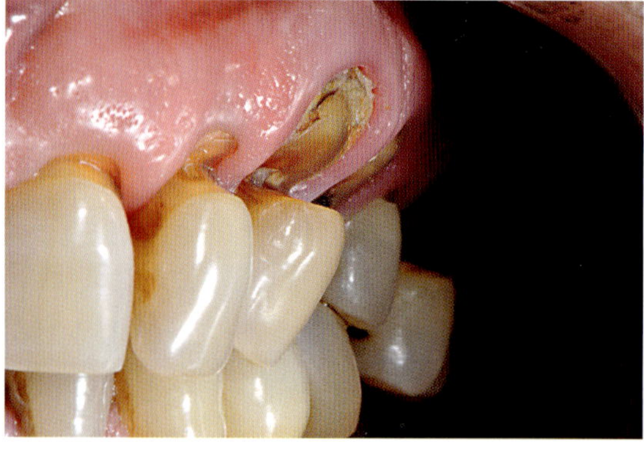

Fig. 2. Multiple root caries associated with advanced periodontal disease.

with untreated caries and restored root surface lesions, especially in persons over 45 years [8]. Post-radiation and xerostomic patients also seem to be at risk for the development of root caries [9].

Although the etiology of root caries and NCCLs are different, both types of lesions are very common, mainly in the elderly, and they are restored similarly. Due to the scarce literature about the treatment of root caries [10] when compared to NCCLs, we will guide the description of the treatment and clinical performance of restorations placed in root caries based on the literature about restoration of NCCLs and the few clinical trials performed in root caries.

Restorative Materials for Clinical Management of Cervical Lesions

Cervical lesions can be restored with composite resins or glass ionomer cements (GIC) or even with both materials, with GIC working as a liner in the so-called sandwich technique. The choice of material for the treatment of root caries and NCCLs depends mainly on the aesthetic involvement, patient's expectations and needs, as well as the caries activity of the patient.

Resin composite materials may produce in most of the cases imperceptible restorations; while GIC is highly opaque contrasting with the dental structure, which makes it harder to produce aesthetic restorations with GIC. Resin-modified GICs (RMGIC) are more aesthetic than GIC, but inferior to resin composite materials.

On the contrary, GIC and RMGIC have the ability to deliver fluorides [11] to the dental structures and neighboring teeth, which is of great importance when dealing with caries-active patients due to its continuing action through time [12]. Additionally, both types of GIC are self-adhesive materials and in principle do not require any surface pre-treatment. In some cases, pre-treatment with polyalkenoic acid may improve the adhesion of these materials with the dental structure by removing the most superficial smear layer.

Resin composites need pre-treatment with adhesive systems. Nowadays, there are etch-and-rinse adhesives (ER), self-etch adhesives (SE), and universal adhesive systems. The degree of substance exchange substantially differs among these adhesives. In general, the exchange intensity induced by ER adhesives exceeds that of SE adhesives, though among the latter, there are systems that intensively interact with tooth tissue [13].

In general, we can say that ER systems are available in 2 or 3 clinical steps, the first step being the application of a *conditioner* or acid etchant. This conditioner (commonly phosphoric-acid

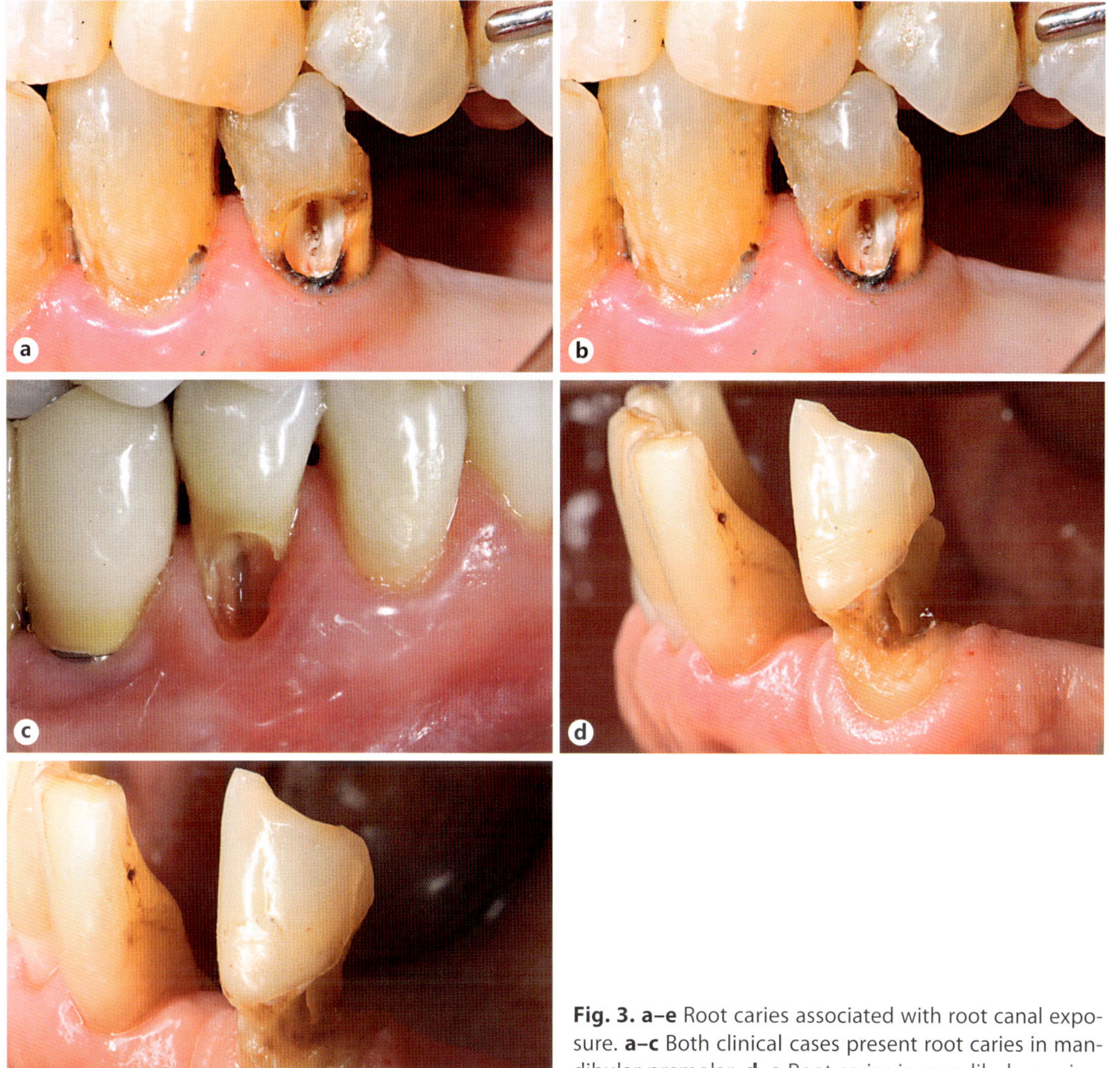

Fig. 3. a–e Root caries associated with root canal exposure. **a–c** Both clinical cases present root caries in mandibular premolar. **d**, **e** Root caries in mandibular canine. Observe the irregular aspect of lesion after contaminated dentin removal.

gel) produces selective dissolution of enamel and dentin. In dentin, this procedure exposes a collagen layer free of minerals, which is readily filled with resin monomers. After in situ polymerization of resin monomers, resin tags within the dentin tubules and a hybrid layer is created providing micromechanical retention and sealing. When the adhesive application is done in 3 steps, the adhesives are named 3-step ER systems and when in 2 steps, they are named 2-step ER systems (simplified ER system) [13].

On the contrary, SE systems do not require the application of a pre-conditioner rinsing. It no longer needs an "etch-and-rinse" phase, which not only lessens clinical application time, but also significantly reduces technique-sensitivity or the risk of making errors during application and manipulation [13]. In SE adhesives, infiltration of

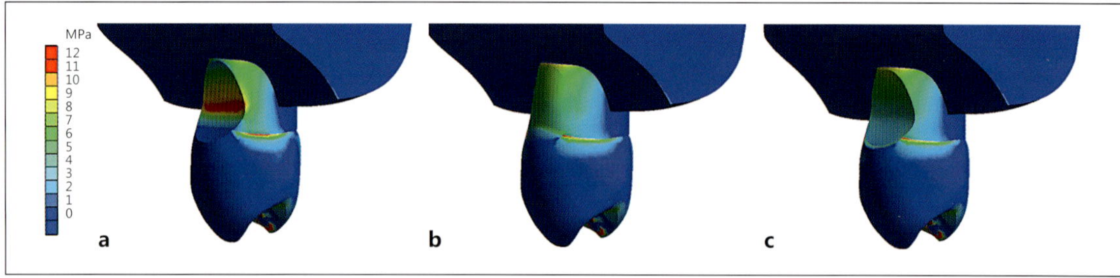

Fig. 4. 3D-Finite Element Analysis of maxillary premolar with root caries. **a** von Mises criteria was applied to show high stress concentration in caries lesion. It means that the cavity created by root caries can promote mechanical stress concentration, which can collaborate on lesion evolution. **b** Composite resin simulation and (**c**) view of the dentin below the composite resin restoration. Observe that adhesive restorations favor mechanical stress distribution and reduce the evolution process of root caries.

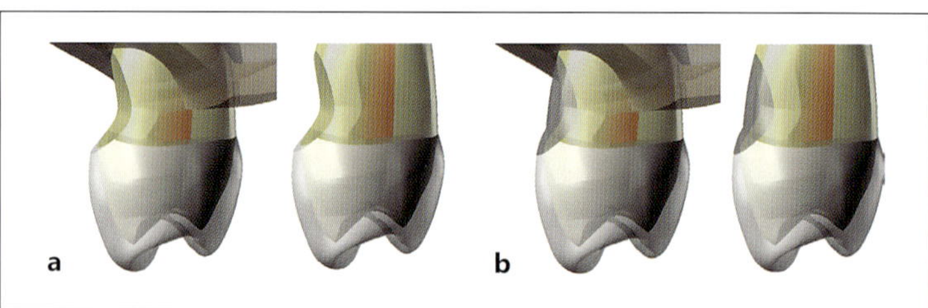

Fig. 5. a 3D virtual models to simulate root caries on maxillary premolar and (**b**) composite restoration.

resin occurs simultaneously with the self-etching process that creates a thinner hybrid layer than the ER protocol. This bonding strategy can be performed in 2 steps (2-step SE) or in a single step (1-step SE). Yet, we still have universal adhesives. In essence, they are mild 1-step self-etch systems that can be used with or without a preliminary rinsing conditioning step.

We cannot deny that the clinical effectiveness of root cervical restorations depends on the type of restorative material chosen and the type of adhesive system selected for resin composites. Root caries can promote deep dentin removal and create cavities of several morphologies. Root caries occurs in important mechanical region of tooth: cervical region, which in most cases coincide with the fulcrum region. The fulcrum region presents high mechanical stress concentration under occlusal load application. The stress concentration may contribute to caries lesion evolution. Many technologies can be used to show this factor, for example, 3D Finite Element Analysis (Fig. 4, 5).

The restoration of cervical lesions with adhesives promote better stress distribution of the masticatory forces at the cervical area and may reduce further wear of the dental structure (Fig. 4, 5). In the following sections, we will describe some important aspects of the clinical procedures used to restore cervical lesions, based on evidence-based findings to guide clinicians' decisions in their clinical practices (Table 1).

Important Issues for Restorations of Cervical Lesions

Resin-Based Composites versus GICs

Many randomized clinical trials (RCTs) have performed this comparison, which allowed the

Table 1. Clinical decisions and strategies that improve or may improve the retention and marginal discoloration of restorations in cervical lesions

Strategies that may improve restoration quality and retention, but still deserve further investigations	Strategies that improve retention, based on available literature
Dentin roughening	Use of GIC instead of composite resins
Use of MMP-inhibitors after acid etching for ER adhesives	Use of partial caries removal or complete removal does not affect GIC retention
Enamel beveling	Active (vigorous) adhesive application (for both SE and ER adhesives) Increase in the number of adhesive coats (SE and ER) Placement of a hydrophobic coating in one-step SE adhesives Dentin pre-treatment with EDTA for SE adhesives Selective enamel etching for SE adhesives

MMP, Matrix metalloproteinase; ER, etch-and-rinse; GIC, glass ionomer cements; SE, self-etch; EDTA, ethylenediaminetetraacetic acid.

conduction of a systematic review with a meta-analysis, by our research group. We observed that the 3-year retention rates of RMGIC were 76% higher than that observed with resin-based composites. In the 5-year comparison, the retention rate of the RMGIC was 87% higher than resin-based composites. Our findings are in agreement with a systematic review [14] that concluded that GIC has a significantly lower risk of restoration loss than resin-based composite resins placed with a 3-step ER and 2-step ER systems. However, difficulties to match the dental color are likely responsible for the reduced use of RMGI in these types of lesions.

Minimal Intervention for Removal of Root Caries Lesions

Some studies have investigated whether or not the removal of caries lesions following a conventional treatment or using atraumatic restorative approach (ART) would affect the retention rates of restorations placed in root caries lesions [15–19]. ART is an alternative technique in which the softened tissue of the lesion is removed with a manual instrument and is sealed with an adhesive, such as GIC. ART takes the advantage of being more conservative, painless, and executable in environments without dental offices.

Most of these studies conclude that the retention rates of GIC and RMGIC restorations placed in cervical lesions with the ART protocol do not differ compared to those that followed conventional methods for caries removal [15, 16, 18]. Additionally, another study did not find evidence that the use of an enzymatic gel (Carisolv) for caries removal affect the retention rates of cervical restorations [20].

Rubber Dam versus Cotton Rolls/Retraction Cord Isolation

Two recent low-sample sized clinical trials that evaluated the effect of type of isolation method on the performance of resin composite restoration in cervical lesions did not find any evidence that supports a superiority of one technique over the other [21, 22]. This was also supported by 2 other systematic reviews [23, 24]. Regardless of the type of isolation method chosen, the operative field should be clean, dry, free of saliva and crevicular fluid contamination as these factors may reduce the bonding of adhesive systems with the dental surface [25, 26].

Cavity Preparation

When dealing with root caries, the carious lesion should be removed using conventional techniques (burs) or using minimally invasive approaches (instrument manual removal), as adhesion to caries-affected dentin is lower than sound dentin [27, 28]. The type of caries removal did not affect the retention rates of these restorations [15, 16, 18].

In case of NCCLs, doubts about whether or not to perform *dentin roughening* to remove the most superficial and mineralized sclerotic dentin layer arise. Although some clinical trials have attempted to evaluate this issue [29], they found no evidence of difference among techniques. On the contrary, other systematic reviews that performed indirect correlation between some protocol variations and the retention rates of NCCLs found that dental roughening are associated with increased retention rates [23, 24]. However, the evidence produced by the 2 latter systematic reviews indirectly reduces the quality of the evidence and should be still interpreted with caution. There is still room for the conduction of further RCTs, with a rigorous methodology, to evaluate this issue.

Enamel beveling is another clinical question. No RCT that investigated this issue found higher retention rates of composite resins when enamel beveling was placed [24, 30, 31]. In a recent systematic review, Schroeder concluded that by evaluating studies with low risk of bias we cannot state that enamel beveling improves the retention rates of resin-composites in cervical lesions [32]. However, from our clinical experience, it seems easier to hide the interface between resin composite and the dental cavity when enamel beveling is performed, but this is not unanimous among clinicians [33].

Application of the Adhesive System Prior to Resin Composite Placement

As bonding interfaces are highly prone to degradation due to the plasticization of resin monomers that infiltrates into the demineralized dentin matrix and due to enzymatic attack of exposed collagen fibrils by endogenous host-derived enzymes [34], several in vitro studies have attempted to investigate bonding techniques to improve the durability of dentin interfaces.

As a rule of thumb, adhesive systems should be applied following manufacturer's instructions. However, some RCTs showed that changes in the clinical protocol (described below) may yield better clinical performance, such as higher retention rates and lower marginal discoloration. In the following section of the chapter, we will only report the approaches that were clinically investigated. More details about other techniques can be found in another publication [34].

Active Adhesive Application

Regardless of the adhesive systems employed, active adhesive application can increase the 2-year retention rates of resin composite restorations placed in NCCLs [35], as it improves monomer infiltration, demineralization of the dentin substrate (in case of SE adhesives), and more outward diffusion of solvent. This clinical step is so important that it reduces the importance of the "wet bonding technique" when using ER adhesives [36]. A clinical study reported that as long as adhesives are applied vigorously, adhesives can be applied in a dry or wet condition as the moisture of dentin does not affect the 2-year retention rates of ER adhesives [36]. The active application should preferably be performed with a rigid microbrush rather than bristle-like applicators.

Increase in the Number of Adhesive Coats

Increasing the number of adhesive coats, mainly for a single-step SE, resulted in higher retention rates [37, 38] than those achieved following the manufacturer's instructions. It is likely that the additional layers of adhesive may improve the etching ability of SE adhesives and increase their impregnation into the dental substrates.

Placement of Hydrophobic Resin Coating in One-Step SE Adhesives

This is especially important for 1-step SE adhesives. As previously mentioned, adhesives are prone to degradation over time and this seems to be directly correlated with the hydrophilicity of the adhesive composition [27, 28]. One-step SE are, among all adhesive classes, the one with more hydrophilic features, placing them (as there are exceptions) at a higher risk of failure [39]. For some of them, the placement of an additional hydrophobic layer makes them less hydrophilic, and this approach can lead to increased retention rates of composite restorations in cervical lesions [40]. However, the high variability of the compositions of 1-step SE adhesives [41, 42] explains why a rigorous systematic review did not gather evidence that one adhesive strategy is better than the other [43].

Use of Matrix Metalloproteinase-Inhibitor after Dentin Acid Etching

Laboratory findings have demonstrated that the application of matrix metalloproteinase-inhibitors (2% chlorhexidine [CHX] for 2 min) on dentin after acid etching may reduce the degradation of the collagen fibrils within the hybrid layer. However, the available short clinical studies on this issue have not found any evidence that this procedure improves or jeopardizes the retention rates of NCCLs [44], even when CHX was incorporated into the composition of an adhesive system [45]. Therefore, whether or not we use it during clinical bonding is a clinicians' decision. Further long-term RCTs are needed to clarify whether CHX may sustain an antiproteolytic activity as it has demonstrated in vitro studies.

Dentin Pre-Treatment for SE Adhesives

EDTA application (17% EDTA for 2 min) before the use of an SE adhesive [46] improved the 18-month retention rates of restorations, probably by providing a mild demineralization of the sclerotic dentin and exposing a more reactive dentin layer for the demineralization and infiltration of acidic resin monomers from SE adhesives.

Selective Enamel Etching for SE Adhesives

Laboratory findings report that SE adhesives do not etch enamel as well as phosphoric acid [47] as they produce a very shallow enamel etching, with reduced micro-porosities for resin infiltration [47]. This led to reduced bond strength and implies lower retention rates and/or higher marginal discoloration. A recent systematic review about this clinical approach, observed in the meta-analyses of follow-up periods of 2, 3, and 5 years, improved the marginal discoloration and marginal adaptation when selective enamel etching was performed [48]. Additionally, this procedure also improved the 3-year retention rates of the resin-based composite restorations. The micro-retentive and selective etching pattern produced on enamel by phosphoric acid etching likely improved the demineralization and infiltration of the resin monomers from the SE adhesives.

Other Important Issues

Which Adhesive Should be Selected For Resin-Based Composite Restorations?

There are some systematic reviews of the literature that examined the retention rates of adhesives that belong to different adhesive strategies. In 2005, Peumans et al. [39] reported less favorable clinical performance of simplified adhesives (1-step SE and 2-step ER) when compared to the less simplified versions of these strategies (2-step SE and 3-step ER), which is also in agreement with the findings of Heintze et al. [24].

However, more recently, Peumans et al. [42] concluded differently from their earlier review [39]. They reported that the most recent 1-step SE may reach the same clinical performance of 2-step SE and 3-step ER systems. Krithikadatta [49], including studies from 2004 to 2010, concluded that the clinical performance of different categories of more recent bonding systems was comparable.

In the systematic review of Chee et al. [43], by applying a more rigorous selection criteria and robust quality assessment of the primary included RCTs, the authors concluded that in general, studies were not of sufficient quality to allow generalization that a bonding strategy is better than the other [50]. The authors of this chapter suppose that the performance of resin-based composite restoration placed in NCCLs is much more dependable on the balanced chemistry of the material than the bonding strategy employed. Indeed, Chee et al. [43] observed that adhesives evaluated in studies with an overall low risk of bias demonstrated good clinical performance in all 4 bonding strategies.

Regular or Flowable Resin-Based Composites

As the elastic modulus of flowable composites is lower than regular resin composites, they could flex with the dental structure during masticatory movement, favoring retention of restorations. As there are many RCTs on this topic [51–55], we conducted a systematic review to address this clinical question (unpublished data) and we did not find enough evidence to state that flowable composites have higher retention rates than composites with regular viscosity. Therefore, the choice of resin viscosity for the restoration of NCCLs is a clinician's decision.

Conclusion

Most of what we know from the clinical performance of restorations placed in root caries comes from studies in NCCLs. Additionally, the risk of bias of these studies is still high, which reduces the strength of the quality of evidence on this issue. More RCTs with rigorous methodology mainly for root caries should be conducted.

References

1 Kumara-Raja B, Radha G: Prevalence of root caries among elders living in residential homes of Bengaluru city, India. J Clin Exp Dent 2016;8:e260–e267.

2 Bharateesh JV, Kokila G: Association of root caries with oral habits in older individuals attending a rural health centre of a dental hospital in India. J Clin Diagn Res 2014;8:ZC80–ZC82.

3 Imazato S, Ikebe K, Nokubi T, Ebisu S, Walls AW: Prevalence of root caries in a selected population of older adults in Japan. J Oral Rehabil 2006;33:137–143.

4 Watanabe MG: Root caries prevalence in a group of Brazilian adult dental patients. Braz Dent J 2003;14:153–156.

5 Lai ZY, Zhi QH, Zhou Y, Lin HC: Prevalence of non-carious cervical lesions and associated risk indicators in middle-aged and elderly populations in Southern China. Chin J Dent Res 2015;18:41–50.

6 Kumar S, Kumar A, Debnath N, Kumar A, K Badiyani B, Basak D, S A Ali M, B Ismail M: Prevalence and risk factors for non-carious cervical lesions in children attending special needs schools in India. J Oral Sci 2015;57:37–43.

7 Jiang H, Du MQ, Huang W, Peng B, Bian Z, Tai BJ: The prevalence of and risk factors for non-carious cervical lesions in adults in Hubei Province, China. Community Dent Health 2011;28:22–28.

8 Christensen LB, Bardow A, Ekstrand K, Fiehn NE, Heitmann BL, Qvist V, Twetman S: Root caries, root surface restorations and lifestyle factors in adult Danes. Acta Odontol Scand 2015;73:467–473.

9 Cautley AJ: Root caries: some clinical aspects. N Z Dent J 1993;89:132–136.

10 Hayes M, Brady P, Burke FM, Allen PF: Failure rates of class V restorations in the management of root caries in adults – a systematic review. Gerodontology 2016;33:299–307.

11 Eichmiller FC, Marjenhoff WA: Fluoride-releasing dental restorative materials. Oper Dent 1998;23:218–228.

12 Shiiya T, Mukai Y, Ten Cate JM, Teranaka T: The caries-reducing benefit of fluoride-release from dental restorative materials continues after fluoride-release has ended. Acta Odontol Scand 2012;70:15–20.

13 Van Meerbeek B, De Munck J, Yoshida Y, Inoue S, Vargas M, Vijay P, Van Landuyt K, Lambrechts P, Vanherle G: Buonocore memorial lecture. Adhesion to enamel and dentin: current status and future challenges. Oper Dent 2003;28:215–235.

14 Santos MJ, Ari N, Steele S, Costella J, Banting D: Retention of tooth-colored restorations in non-carious cervical lesions – a systematic review. Clin Oral Investig 2014;18:1369–1381.

15 Hu JY, Chen XC, Li YQ, Smales RJ, Yip KH: Radiation-induced root surface caries restored with glass-ionomer cement placed in conventional and ART cavity preparations: results at two years. Aust Dent J 2005;50:186–190.
16 Lo EC, Luo Y, Tan HP, Dyson JE, Corbet EF: ART and conventional root restorations in elders after 12 months. J Dent Res 2006;85:929–932.
17 Cruz Gonzalez AC, Marin Zuluaga DJ: Clinical outcome of root caries restorations using ART and rotary techniques in institutionalized elders. Braz Oral Res 2016;30:pii: S1806-83242016000100260.
18 Steele J: ART for treating root caries in older people. Evid Based Dent 2007;8: 51.
19 Gilboa I, Cardash HS, Baharav H, Demko CA, Teich ST: A longitudinal study of the survival of interproximal root caries lesions restored with glass ionomer cement via a minimally invasive approach. Gen Dent 2012;60:e224–e230.
20 Gil-Montoya JA, Mateos-Palacios R, Bravo M, Gonzalez-Moles MA, Pulgar R: Atraumatic restorative treatment and Carisolv use for root caries in the elderly: 2-year follow-up randomized clinical trial. Clin Oral Investig 2014;18:1089–1095.
21 Daudt E, Lopes GC, Vieira LC: Does operatory field isolation influence the performance of direct adhesive restorations? J Adhes Dent 2013;15:27–32.
22 Loguercio AD, Luque-Martinez I, Lisboa AH, Higashi C, Queiroz VA, Rego RO, Reis A: Influence of isolation method of the operative field on gingival damage, patients' preference, and restoration retention in noncarious cervical lesions. Oper Dent 2015;40:581–593.
23 Mahn E, Rousson V, Heintze S: Meta-analysis of the influence of bonding parameters on the clinical outcome of tooth-colored cervical restorations. J Adhes Dent 2015;17:391–403.
24 Heintze SD, Ruffieux C, Rousson V: Clinical performance of cervical restorations – a meta-analysis. Dent Mater 2010;26:993–1000.
25 Santschi K, Peutzfeldt A, Lussi A, Flury S: Effect of salivary contamination and decontamination on bond strength of two one-step self-etching adhesives to dentin of primary and permanent teeth. J Adhes Dent 2015;17:51–57.
26 Yoo HM, Pereira PN: Effect of blood contamination with 1-step self-etching adhesives on microtensile bond strength to dentin. Oper Dent 2006;31:660–665.
27 Shibata S, Vieira LC, Baratieri LN, Fu J, Hoshika S, Matsuda Y, Sano H: Evaluation of microtensile bond strength of self-etching adhesives on normal and caries-affected dentin. Dent Mater J 2016;35:166–173.
28 Nakajima M, Sano H, Urabe I, Tagami J, Pashley DH: Bond strengths of single-bottle dentin adhesives to caries-affected dentin. Oper Dent 2000;25:2–10.
29 van Dijken JW: Durability of three simplified adhesive systems in Class V noncarious cervical dentin lesions. Am J Dent 2004;17:27–32.
30 Perdigao J, Carmo AR, Anauate-Netto C, Amore R, Lewgoy HR, Cordeiro HJ, Dutra-Correa M, Castilhos N: Clinical performance of a self-etching adhesive at 18 months. Am J Dent 2005;18:135–140.
31 Baratieri LN, Canabarro S, Lopes GC, Ritter AV: Effect of resin viscosity and enamel beveling on the clinical performance of Class V composite restorations: three-year results. Oper Dent 2003;28:482–487.
32 Schroeder M, Reis A, Luque-Martinez I, Loguercio AD, Masterson D, Maia LC: Effect of enamel bevel on retention of cervical composite resin restorations: a systematic review and meta-analysis. J Dent 2015;43:777–788.
33 Baratieri LN, Ritter AV: Critical appraisal. To bevel or not in anterior composites. J Esthet Restor Dent 2005;17:264–269.
34 Reis A, Carrilho M, Breschi L, Loguercio AD: Overview of clinical alternatives to minimize the degradation of the resin-dentin bonds. Oper Dent 2013;38:E1–E25.
35 Loguercio AD, Raffo J, Bassani F, Balestrini H, Santo D, do Amaral RC, Reis A: 24-month clinical evaluation in non-carious cervical lesions of a two-step etch-and-rinse adhesive applied using a rubbing motion. Clin Oral Investig 2011; 15:589–596.
36 Zander-Grande C, Amaral RC, Loguercio AD, Barroso LP, Reis A: Clinical performance of one-step self-etch adhesives applied actively in cervical lesions: 24-month clinical trial. Oper Dent 2014; 39:228–238.
37 Loguercio AD, Reis A: Application of a dental adhesive using the self-etch and etch-and-rinse approaches: an 18-month clinical evaluation. J Am Dent Assoc 2008;139:53–61.
38 Loguercio AD, Costenaro A, Silveira AP, Ribeiro NR, Rossi TR, Reis A: A six-month clinical study of a self-etching and an etch-and-rinse adhesive applied as recommended and after doubling the number of adhesive coats. J Adhes Dent 2006;8:255–261.
39 Peumans M, Kanumilli P, De Munck J, Van Landuyt K, Lambrechts P, Van Meerbeek B: Clinical effectiveness of contemporary adhesives: a systematic review of current clinical trials. Dent Mater 2005;21:864–881.
40 Reis A, Leite TM, Matte K, Michels R, Amaral RC, Geraldeli S, Loguercio AD: Improving clinical retention of one-step self-etching adhesive systems with an additional hydrophobic adhesive layer. J Am Dent Assoc 2009;140:877–885.
41 Van Landuyt KL, Snauwaert J, De Munck J, Peumans M, Yoshida Y, Poitevin A, Coutinho E, Suzuki K, Lambrechts P, Van Meerbeek B: Systematic review of the chemical composition of contemporary dental adhesives. Biomaterials 2007;28:3757–3785.
42 Peumans M, De Munck J, Mine A, Van Meerbeek B: Clinical effectiveness of contemporary adhesives for the restoration of non-carious cervical lesions. A systematic review. Dent Mater 2014;30: 1089–1103.
43 Chee B, Rickman LJ, Satterthwaite JD: Adhesives for the restoration of non-carious cervical lesions: a systematic review. J Dent 2012;40:443–452.
44 Montagner AF, Perroni AP, Correa MB, Masotti AS, Pereira-Cenci T, Cenci MS: Effect of pre-treatment with chlorhexidine on the retention of restorations: a randomized controlled trial. Braz Dent J 2015;26:234–241.
45 Araujo MS, Souza LC, Apolonio FM, Barros LO, Reis A, Loguercio AD, Saboia VP: Two-year clinical evaluation of chlorhexidine incorporation in two-step self-etch adhesive. J Dent 2015;43:140–148.
46 Luque-Martinez I, Munoz MA, Mena-Serrano A, Hass V, Reis A, Loguercio AD: Effect of EDTA conditioning on cervical restorations bonded with a self-etch adhesive: A randomized double-blind clinical trial. J Dent 2015;43:1175–1183.

47 Moura SK, Pelizzaro A, Dal Bianco K, de Goes MF, Loguercio AD, Reis A, Grande RH: Does the acidity of self-etching primers affect bond strength and surface morphology of enamel? J Adhes Dent 2006;8:75–83.

48 Szesz A, Parreiras S, Reis A, Loguercio A: Selective enamel etching in cervical lesions for self-etch adhesives: a systematic review and meta-analysis. J Dent 2016;53:1–11.

49 Krithikadatta J: Clinical effectiveness of contemporary dentin bonding agents. J Conserv Dent 2010;13:173–183.

50 Pendrys DG: Existing evidence is not sufficient to accept or refute the superiority of any adhesive system for the restoration of non-carious cervical lesions. J Evid Based Dent Pract 2012;12:196–198.

51 Boeckler A, Schaller HG, Gernhardt CR: A prospective, double-blind, randomized clinical trial of a one-step, self-etch adhesive with and without an intermediary layer of a flowable composite: a 2-year evaluation. Quintessence Int 2012;43:279–286.

52 Celik EU, Aka B, Yilmaz F: Six-month clinical evaluation of a self-adhesive flowable composite in noncarious cervical lesions. J Adhes Dent 2015;17:361–368.

53 Stefanski S, van Dijken JW: Clinical performance of a nanofilled resin composite with and without an intermediary layer of flowable composite: a 2-year evaluation. Clin Oral Investig 2012;16:147–153.

54 Efes BG, Dorter C, Gomec Y, Koray F: Two-year clinical evaluation of ormocer and nanofill composite with and without a flowable liner. J Adhes Dent 2006;8:119–126.

55 Gallo JR, Burgess JO, Ripps AH, Walker RS, Maltezos MB, Mercante DE, Davidson JM: Three-year clinical evaluation of two flowable composites. Quintessence Int 2010;41:497–503.

Prof. Alessandra Reis
Departamento de Odontologia, Universidade Estadual de Ponta Grossa
Av. Carlos Cavalcanti, 4748 – Bloco M
Ponta Grossa, PR 84030-900 (Brazil)
E-Mail reis_ale@hotmail.com

Carrilho MRO (ed): Root Caries: From Prevalence to Therapy.
Monogr Oral Sci. Basel, Karger, 2017, vol 26, pp 125–132 (DOI: 10.1159/000479355)

Concluding Remarks

Marcela Rocha de Olivera Carrilho

Anhanguera University of São Paulo, Biomaterials and Biotechnology & Innovation in Health Programs, São Paulo, Brazil

Abstract

Case reports and clinical trials conducted in different countries (i.e., the United States, Canada, Brazil, Germany, Finland, Sweden, Japan, India, and Sri Lanka) tend to find a positive relationship between the presence of more retained teeth in older ages and the prevalence of root caries in older adults. As this tendency has been shown to prevail globally, it is estimated that the predicted demographic elderly expansion may cause, in near future, a significant increment in the number of older population requiring an effective means of preventing and treating root surface caries. Based on these concerns, the editors of the series *Monographs in Oral Science* by Karger Publishers, Dr. Adrian Lussi and Dr. Marilia Buzalaf, have invited me to organize a book, in which it was reunited a team of experts who could provide a critical and comprehensive understanding on the different aspects concurring for the *caries phenomenon* development on dental *root surfaces*. This team effort turned into a superb publication; the different parts of the book are indeed at the top level. Collectively, the chapters of this book brought a wide picture of the state-of-the-art in the addressed themes, which in turn will hopefully serve as a reference for readers and encourage new researches in the area.

This concluding remarks present some closing thoughts on the current knowledge concerning the macro theme *Root Caries*, minutely discussed in this book by a panel of well-recognized and new-talent experts from different parts of the globe. It includes challenges (and learnt lessons) when organizing a book with a fixed guiding theme, especially for a novice like me in this duty. Having come to the end, I now realize that actually the easiest aspect of this endeavor was exactly having this guiding theme, *Root Caries,* as inspirational wellspring. It is insightful to perceive that the improvements in dental care and the current knowledge on caries prevention have contributed, in general terms, to reduce the teeth loss rating for an aging world population in comparison to past generations. Although caries experience has been relatively reduced over the past decades, it keeps figuring, according to the World Health Organization (WHO), among the most prevalent chronic diseases in the world [1].

Keeping due proportions, mainly related to the socioeconomic and/or sociocultural/educational development levels, the world has been witnessing a systematic and continuous increase in the older population globally. In 2015, the adults aged 65 years or over represented 8.5% of the total population (or 617.1 million people) [2]. It is estimated that the older population will almost double to 1.6 billion between 2025 and 2050, whereas the total population will grow by just 34% over the same period [2]. The transition from high to low mortality and fertility also implies a shift in the leading causes of disease and death. Demographers and epidemiologists explain this changeover as part of an "epidemiologic transition" distinguished by the decline of infectious and acute diseases and the emerging significance of chronic and degenerative diseases [3]. As the world population continues to grow older, it has been observed, for instance, that there is an increasing difficulty for this population to effectively control the oral biofilm. Besides, the prevalence of gingival recessions also increases with age, thereby root surfaces are more frequently exposed to the oral environment; consequently, the risk for developing root caries lesions is potentially higher [4–9]. Accordingly, the anticipated demographic elderly boom will probably lead to a large increase in the number of older adults with root caries therapy requirements and a demand for even more effective means of preventing *Root Caries*. In view of these facts, the editors-in-chief of the series *Monographs in Oral Science* by Karger, Dr. Adrian Lussi and Dr. Marilia Buzalaf, along with this series editorial board, have conceived the idea of producing a publication entirely focused on this subject, and invited me to participate in this project as a guest editor.

The first step towards organizing this publication was made by defining the discussion axes, which in turn divided this publication into 4 core parts, so-nominated: *Epidemiology; Biological Determinants; Lesion Assessment and Features,* and *Preventive and Operative Therapies*. With the editors-in-chief's approval, the themes (or chapters) within each discussion axis were then suggested and, finally, a careful search on academic databases and search engines (Pubmed, SciELO, Scopus, EMBASE, Google Scholar) popped up the authors who have been demonstrating a consistent familiarity and scientific background to write down and develop each proposed chapter. The result is an excellent piece of contribution to the correlate literature; and I feel absolutely comfortable with this judgment since I do not figure between authors or co-authors of any chapter. Genuinely, the different parts of this book are at the top level, confirming that the bests were selected and accepted to share their scientific expertise in the requested topics.

As a guest editor, I am very proud with the final outcome of the book. As a reader, I feel thrilled with the approach and new information finely discussed by this great team of collaborators. And finally as a researcher, I assume this book can also be seen as a source of new ideas and hypotheses that could be further investigated in the future. A brief summary of chapters' content is presented as an attempt to highlight the most useful information generously mined and shared by this team of new and well-established experts.

Root Caries: Epidemiology Session

There are now several indicators that provide insight into the incidence and prevalence of caries in healthy people and the medical or disability conditions that place individuals at increased caries risk. The two chapters of this session, both under the responsibility of Dr. Hayes and her collaborators Dr. Burke and Dr. Allen, brought up to discussion the fundamental importance of basing these analyses on high quality epidemiological data since this type of approach guides, when necessary, government and health authorities to enplane national oral health policies with cost-effective targeting of nation's resources. Despite the intrinsic significance provided by epidemiological studies, Hayes et al. (pp. 1–8) argue that due to either scarcity or heterogeneity of clinical studies in this field, it is so far not possible for one to reach a broad conclusion on the global burden of root surface caries. In this chapter, authors also mentioned that the lack of consensus on a definition for root caries, and the considerable debate about how best to measure it, reveal how complicated the epidemiology of this disease is. Finally, this first chapter pointed out that clinical (epidemiological) studies concerning root caries' development and particularities are frequently concentrated on older adults because this seems to be the population mostly affected by this ailment. Taking this into consideration, the second chapter of this publication starts affirming that an increase in exposed root surfaces in the over 65 age group predisposes this group to a higher prevalence of root caries than younger populations. Moreover, here, authors keep paying attention to the fact that the lack of well-defined terminology in the study of root caries leads to challenges in interpreting the reported prevalence and incidence of root caries. They also suggested that root surface may be more vulnerable to mechanical destruction than the crown because the structure and chemical composition of cementum make it more soluble and/or wearable with regard to enamel. So, in a population who are frequently exposed to scaling by dental health professionals, the cementum layer is frequently abraded away, exposing the dentin. Hayes et al. ended up concluding that to count on past root caries experience as a predictor tool of risk assessment for preventive purposes is falling as it precludes the opportunity to identify a high risk for individuals before they become exposed to the disease (pp. 9–14).

Root Caries: Biological Determinants Session

Determinant factors of dental root surface caries could be envisaged from many levels, and whether or not root caries is a unique physiopathological entity, it certainly depends on the biological scale being considered. Likewise, the biological determinants of root caries could also be examined under different prospects. In this session, the biological aspects discussed as playing a decisive role for root incidence were: *Biofilm, Saliva, Gingival Fluid and Endogenous enzymes.* Dr. Damé-Teixeira and her collaborators Dr. Parolo and Dr. Maltz, opened up this session addressing in overall terms the specificities of caries on root surface. This chapter "Specificities of Caries on Root Surface" (pp. 15–25) reinforced the notion that variations in organic and inorganic compositions and morphology may determine different susceptibilities of root surfaces to caries when compared to coronal surface. Special attention was given on revisiting the biochemical, structural, and histopathological specificities of root caries. Among several conclusions, the authors stated that tissues forming the dental root and periodontal structures have singular characteristics in terms of composition and anatomy, which may change their response to different cariogenic challenges. In sequence, the chapter led by Dr. Do with fine collaboration of Dr. Damé-Teixeira, Dr. Naginyte, and Dr. Marsh consisted of a fascinating and up-to-date review on the contribution of biofilm, saliva, and gingival fluid to the physiopathology of root caries. The bottom line of this chapter assumed that saliva and gingival crevicular fluid actually affect the composition of biofilms which are developed on the root surface. Moreover, this chapter highlighted that the main sources of nutrients for the microorganisms attached to the root surface are the proteins and glycoproteins present in saliva and gingival crevicular fluid. Finally, the authors mentioned that the acquired pellicle on exposed root surfaces contains more plasma proteins compared to enamel, and these may influence the pattern of biofilm formation. Dr. Chaussain and her colleagues Dr. Boukpessi and Dr. Menashi wrote another quite motivating chapter ("Endogenous Enzymes in Root Caries", pp. 35–42) about the role of endogenous enzymes in the development of root caries lesions. They emphasized that similar to coronal caries, the demineralization and exposure of the root dentin or cementum organic matrix by acid production from cariogenic bacteria may induce the activation of endogenous (host-derived) enzymes within the dentin and saliva. Then, the state-of-art concerning the expression and activity of host-derived enzymes, matrix metalloproteases and cystein proteases (cathepsins), present either in dentin or saliva, were reviewed with regard to their contribution to caries lesion progression. Finally, authors conclude that in contrast to coronal caries where dentin is protected by enamel, root caries progress more rapidly due to the salivary matrix metalloproteases, which have a direct access to the matrix-organic mineralized dental tissues. Thus, this may easily initiate the degradation process once the cementum or dentin surface is demineralized by bacterial acids.

Root Caries: Lesion Assessment Session

Several conferences were held over the past decades with the intention of discussing and establishing criteria for caries detection and management. Since the last consensus on Diagnosis and Management of Dental Caries held in 2002 [10], not much has changed considerably (or differently reported) in terms of caries lesion assessment recommendation. In this session of the series, a cast of experienced authors has undertaken to revisit the general terms related to this topic as well as present a critical analysis on the concept definitions and methods currently available to access and control caries lesions. In the chapter written by Dr. Fejerskov and Dr. Nyvad, two of the most important authorities when talking about caries detection and management, give us a quite remarkable design on the rationale behind the good practices for achieving an effective diagnosis of root caries. They reminded that diagnosing and choosing appropriate treatment for root surface caries requires basic knowledge of the clinical appearance and histopathology of the disease. Then, they also emphasized that for purposes of treatment decision, root caries lesions should first be classified into "active" or "inactive" lesions. According to the authors, such a distinction would be useful in recording the oral health status of the individual, as it gives an immediate impression of previous caries challenges as well as an indication of the need for active professional intervention and caries control at the time of examination. Among other helpful hints, Dr. Fejerskov and Dr. Nyvad ended up concluding that the poor prognosis of operative treatment of root surface caries indicates that operative treatment should be avoided as much as possible in favor of non-operative caries control strategies. The following chapter under the responsibility of other two experienced authors in the subject, Dr. Doméjean and Dr. Banerjee, dedicates its attention to the principle that the ability to assess a patient's susceptibility to developing root surface carious lesions accurately is indeed crucial for the determination and implementation of appropriate patient-focused preventive strategies, hence resulting in perhaps reduced need for complex operative treatments and associated morbidity. This chapter points out that, among the variety of caries susceptibility/risk assessment protocols, only CAMBRA (caries management by risk assessment) and ADA (caries risk assessment and management by the American Dental Association) methods consider the criterion "exposed roots" to be accounted for to get a logical systematic approach to synthesizing information about caries disease. Conversely, even if such a criterion is included in these 2 protocols, it does not do so with the intention to assess the specific risk for root caries development but actually to assess the overall patient susceptibility to develop carious lesions, whatever the surface. Thus, the authors finally concluded that although the literature may discuss the different factors related to root caries experience, so far there is no model or system to specifically assess the risk for one to develop carious lesions on root surfaces. Dr. Carvalho and Dr. Lussi (editor-in-chief of this series) were among the early birds of this publication, having sent their chapter ("Assessment of Root Caries Lesion Activity and Its Histopathological Features", pp. 63–69) one day before the original estimated deadline! As experts on the assessment of caries activity criteria, they prepared a great text, driving readers to understand how specific histological features of root caries lesions may influence the assessment of lesions activity. It emphasized that since caries lesions result from a dynamic demineralization and remineralization process, it is possible to observe, within the same lesion, areas of active caries, areas of inactive caries, as well as areas of remineralization, aspects which thus illustrate the difficulty in distinguishing between lesions in the initial stages of inactivation (remineralizing) and lesions that still sustain active demineralization. It was also pondered that once the lesions are actually inactive, they present some specific histological aspects easier to recognize. Then, it might be concluded that, in short, inactive lesions are hard, and lie within some distance from the gingival margin, while, in contrast, active lesions are soft/leathery, and found close to the gingival margin. Finally, the authors reckoned that the assessment of lesion activity should be mainly based on tactile sensation and position of the lesion with respect to the gingival margin. This session is closed with the chapter by Dr. Pretty ("Monitoring of Root Caries Lesions", pp. 70–75, who accepted to contribute for this publication even though having a shorter deadline to do so. This happened because, after having received the other chapters of this session, I realized it would be important to include some information on the available approaches/methods to monitor root caries lesions. So, this chapter started underlining the importance of early detection of root caries to the implementation of appropriate and successful preventive therapeutic regimes. Despite this ponderation, Dr. Pretty also showed evidences that the detection of early root caries can be more complex than that of enamel caries as the early white spot lesion seen on the latter, is not present on the former. Moreover, Dr. Pretty presented and discussed the scoring system proposed by Ekstrand et al. [11] to determine root caries activity; and pondered that although the combination of hardness, location, cavitation, and shine are the predominant indicators of both the presence and status of root caries lesions, there are critical issues when recognizing such features within clinical records that complicate the process of longitudinal monitoring of such lesions. In this sense, according to this chapter conclusions, the electronic monitor caries methods such as optical and laser-based systems would offer future potential to enhance the recognition of early root caries for preventive and arrestment purposes.

Root Caries: Preventive and Operative Therapies Session

Prevention and intervention strategies for medical and oral health care have been increasingly designed upon clinical decision-making approaches that require an integration of systemic assessments of clinically scientific evidences concerning the patient's systemic and local condition and history, the practitioner expertise, and the patient's treatment necessities and compliance. The final session of this book is dedicated to discussing the preventive and operative therapies currently available to intervene in the control, arrest, and/or restoration of root caries lesions. As the non-operative intervention seems to be always preferable over the operative ones when controlling/arresting caries, in general (see Fejerskov and Nyvad, pp. 43–54), 4 out of 6 chapters of this session addressed comments and concepts about techniques and resources indicated to interrupt caries progression and/or act as an adjuvant for its control without using restorative biomaterials. The first chapter of this session led by Dr. Maltz with co-authorship of Dr. Alves and Dr. Zenkner focuses on the role of biofilm control and oral hygiene practices in the management of dental caries (pp. 76–82). They made a revision of the most relevant laboratory and clinical (epidemiological or not) studies that had such practices (biofilm control and/or oral hygiene) as the main analyzed factor contributing to root caries arrestment. The authors recognized a bias factor in the studies' results likely attributed to the fact that, in most cases, toothbrushing was usually performed using fluoride-containing agents. The well-known effects of fluorides on caries management make it difficult to isolate the role of self-performed biofilm control in the conservative treatment of carious lesions. Despite such critical point of revised studies, this chapter reunited a number of other evidences to confirm that adequate oral hygiene is of utmost importance in the prevention of root caries, not solely by mechanical biofilm control, but also when aided by the use of fluorides. Taking this last topic into deeper consideration, in chapter by Dr. Magalhães ("Conventional Preventive Therapies (Fluoride) on Root Caries Lesions", pp. 83–87), she reviewed the literature concerning the effects of fluorides (self-applied and professional products) on the prevention and control of root surface caries (pp. 83–87). She showed that, in concert, some clinical trials conducted during 6–8 months with elder people, including disabled nursing home residents, tend to demonstrate that high concentrated fluoride toothpastes (5,000 ppm F) could significantly arrest root caries (by hardness analysis) when compared to conventional toothpastes containing 1,350–1,450 ppm F. In addition, it is mentioned that silver diamond fluoride solution/varnish and NaF varnish are the most often professional-applied products tested for root caries control; with silver diamine fluoride being apparently more advantageous when the frequency of application is considered. Other reviewed studies put under discussion the combined effect of self-applied and professional products. Concluding, Dr. Magalhães stated that despite some clinical evidence about the efficacy of fluoride on the prevention of root surface caries, there is a gap in the knowledge about the benefit (cost-effectiveness) and the optimal use of professional fluoride application combined with the daily use of fluoride toothpaste. Following, the chapter by Dr. Buzalaf (editor-in-chief of this series) and Dr. Pessan ("New Preventive Approaches Part I: Functional Peptides and Other Therapies to Prevent Tooth Demineralization", pp. 88–96), in view of the positive, but commonly limited effect of fluoride on root caries, sought to approach the use of new preventive therapies such as functional peptides, lasers, and phosphate-based technologies in the management of caries lesions (pp. 88–96). They showed that most of the specific peptides currently investigated have been developed based on the available information related to the protective action of salivary proteins, including statherin-derived peptides. Accordingly, laboratory studies have shown that functional peptides tend to increase remineralization and/or protect dental tissues against demineralization through different mechanisms, including the attraction of calcium ions to the demineralized tissue, delivery of available calcium, and antimicrobial action. Regarding phosphate-based technologies, the addition of polyphosphate salts to fluoridated vehicles has been shown to promote a synergistic effect in enamel remineralization and on the prevention of demineralization either in in vitro, in situ or clinical protocols. In addition, laser therapy has also been shown to have synergistic/additive effects with fluoride on the prevention of root dentin demineralization. Dr. Buzalaf and Dr. Pessan ended up concluding that although all these therapies seem to be promising adjuvants to prevent root caries in future, clinical evidence is still required before they can be broadly recommended for use. In sequence, the next chapter of this session ("New Preventive Approaches Part II: Role of Dentin Biomodifiers in Caries Progression", pp. 97–105) brought another piece of contribution by addressing the potential role of dentin biomodifiers in caries progression. In this chapter, Dr. Bedran-Russo and Dr. Zamperini gave us a general and appealing vision on the rationale behind the use of cross-link agents as tissue biomodifiers that seek for locally enhancing the biological and biomechanical characteristics of tissues, organic matrices by mimicking natural processes. According to this chapter, the primary benefit of biomodifiers in the root caries management would be the biological reinforcement of dentin organic matrix due to direct interactions with dentin collagen. In addition, it is theoretically possible to consider that once densely cross-linked, dentin collagen would offer higher resistance to host-derived enzymatic degradation, including that in caries progression (see Do et al., this volume, pp. 26–34 and Boukpessi et al., this volume, pp. 35–42). In addition, laboratory findings suggested that there are selective biomodifiers agents exhibiting a promising ability to induce remineralization as a calcium nucleator. In conclusion, Dr. Bedran-Russo and Dr. Zamperini have reckoned that in vivo studies are needed to determine clinical effectiveness and applicability of the most promising cross-link agents on the root caries progression. Opening the discussion about the operative therapies currently available to treat root surface caries, Dr. Burrow and his colleague Dr. Stacey made a fine revision on the minimum intervention strategies and alternatives to seal root dentin surface affected by caries (pp. 106–114). The authors take into consideration that when a lesion can be effectively cleaned in conjunction with high fluoride content toothpastes and other remineralizing agents, this should be the treatment of choice. On the contrary, for lesions that are cavitated and cannot be effectively cleaned, the initial management should be to apply remineralizing agents for a period to "harden" lesion margins, thus potentially reducing the prepared cavity and restoration size. They also mentioned that since the restoration site can be easily contaminated, the use of glass ionomer cement (GIC) as restorative biomaterial should be preferable. However, for saliva-deficient patients, resin composite or a combination of resin composite and resin-modified glass ionomer would result in a highly polished, easily cleansable restoration surface that may reduce the potential for further caries initiation. Dr. Burrow and Dr. Stacey finally concluded that the current evidence for the restoration of root caries is poor, thus confirmation on restoration survival and caries risk is still lacking. Scanty outcome about the treatment of root caries is actually the primary motto introduced by Dr. Reis and her co-authors, Dr. Soares, Dr. Geus, and Dr. Loguercio in the ending chapter of this session. Thus, they were led to prepare their chapter by guiding the description of the treatment and clinical performance of restorations placed in root caries based on the literature about restoration of non-carious cervical lesions and the few clinical trials performed in root caries. They argued that although the etiology of root caries and non-carious cervical lesions are different, both types of lesions are very common, mainly in the elderly, and when operative procedures are required for those lesions, they are restored in a similar manner. Then, it was shown that randomized clinical trials tend to indicate that conventional GIC has a significantly lower risk of restoration loss than resin-based composite resins placed with 3-step etch-and-rinse and/or 2-step etch-and-rinse systems. Authors also reviewed some studies that have investigated whether or not the removal of caries lesions following a conventional treatment or using atraumatic restorative approach would affect the retention rates of restorations placed in root caries lesions. Results of these studies indicated that the retention rates of GIC and resin-modified glass ionomer restorations placed in cervical lesions with the atraumatic restorative approach protocol did not differ compared to those that followed conventional methods for caries removal. In addition, this chapter brought out several other useful tips to improve the clinical performance of adhesive restorations, no matter they are prepared on coronal or root surface dentin. Concluding this chapter, Dr. Reis and her colleagues assumed that more randomized clinical trials with rigorous methodology, mainly designed in root caries, are in fact essential for one to reach a consistent opinion on the real effectiveness (and necessity) of restoring these lesions with current available biomaterials.

Acknowledgments

Other than challenging, the experience of editing this book was profoundly pleasing and rewarding for me. I feel honored and grateful for having got invited by Dr. Lussi and Dr. Buzalaf to be a guest editor in this series by Karger, more than a professional opportunity, they gave me all support and full liberty to conceive this book as I wished. I also render immense gratitude to authors and co-authors who have made the best of their efforts, investing their precious time to prepare excellent texts, which are now generously shared with those they might interest. I may mention I am delighted and grateful for Dr. Tjäderhane's Foreword for this book. I am also deeply thankful to Karger Publishers and the team involved in the series *Monographs in Oral Science* for this book organization, edition, production and publication; in special I should thank Nicole Hausmann for her tremendous editorial support, by having contacted authors, sent them reminders, dealt with deadline delays, always with kindness, competence, and extreme respect. At last, I thank Michelangelo Giampaoli, my husband, and my family from whom my free time was temporarily subtracted in order it could be devoted to the organization of this book.

References

1 World Health Organization: Oral Health Fact Sheet N°318, April 2012. http://www.who.int/mediacentre/factsheets/fs318/en/ (assessed June 28, 2017).
2 He W, Goodkind D, Kowal P: in; U.S. Census Bureau, International Population Reports, P95/16-1, An Aging World: 2015. Washington, U.S. Government Publishing Office, 2016.
3 Suzman R, Beard J: Global health and aging: preface. National Institute on Aging website.www.nia.nih.gov/research/publication/global-health-and aging/preface. (accessed June 28, 2017) Published October 2011.
4 Locker D, Slade GD, Leake JL: Prevalence of and factors associated with root decay in older adults in Canada. J Dent Res 1989;68:768–772.
5 Fejerskov O, Baelum V, Ostergaard ES: Root caries in Scandinavia in the 1980s and future trends to be expected in dental caries experience in adults. Adv Dent Res 1993;7:4–14.
6 Wang HY, Petersen PE, Bian JY, Zhang BX: The second national survey of oral health status of children and adults in China. Int Dent J 2002;4:283–290.
7 Gilbert GH, Duncan RP, Dolan TA, Foerster U: Twenty-four month incidence of root caries among a diverse group of adults. Caries Res 2001;35:366–375.
8 Sugihara N, Maki Y, Okawa Y, Hosaka M, Matsukubo T, Takaesu Y: Factors associated with root surface caries in elderly. Bull Tokyo Dent Coll 2010;51:23–30.
9 Kumara-Raja B, Radha G: Prevalence of root caries among elders living in residential homes of Bengaluru city, India. J Clin Exp Dent 2016;8:e260–e267.
10 Pitts NB, Stamm JW: International Consensus Workshop on Caries Clinical Trials (ICW-CCT) – final consensus statements: agreeing where the evidence leads. J Dent Res 2004;83(Spec No C):C125–C128.
11 Ekstrand K, Martignon S, Holm-Pedersen P: Development and evaluation of two root caries controlling programmes for home-based frail people older than 75 years. Gerodontology 2008;25:67–75.

Marcela Rocha de Olivera Carrilho, DDS, PhD
Anhanguera University of São Paulo
Biomaterials and Biotechnology & Innovation in Health Programs
Vila Madalena, Rua Girassol, 584 ap 301A
São Paulo, SP 05433-001 (Brazil)
E-Mail marcelacarrilho@gmail.com

Author Index

Subject Index